Towards a sociology for childhood

Thinking from children's lives

Berry Mayall

Open University Press
Buckingham · Philadelphia

Open University Press
Celtic Court
22 Ballmoor
Buckingham
MK18 1XW

email: enquiries@openup.co.uk
world wide web: www.openup.co.uk

and
325 Chestnut Street
Philadelphia, PA 19106, USA

First Published 2002

A catalogue record of this book is available from the British Library

ISBN   0 335 20842 8 (pb)   0 335 20843 6 (hb)

Library of Congress Cataloging-in-Publication Data
Mayall, Berry.
   Towards a sociology for childhood : thinking from children's lives / Berry
   Mayall.
      p. cm.
   Includes bibliographical references and index.
   ISBN 0-335-20843-6 (hardcover) – ISBN 0-335-20842-8 (pbk.)
   1. Children.   2. Children–Social conditions.   3. Children and adults.
   I. Title.
HQ767.9 .M387 2002
305.23–dc21   2001054507

Typeset by Graphicraft Limited, Hong Kong
Printed in Great Britain by St Edmundsbury Press Ltd, Bury St Edmunds, Suffolk

This book is for children, and among them my grandchildren:
Louis, Alice-Mae and Noah Mayall.

Contents

Acknowledgements

I am grateful to very many people over the years, for their written work and for discussions with them. They include: Leena Alanen, Priscilla Alderson, Gill Bendelow, David Buckingham, Kate Gavron, Suzanne Hood, Fatima Husain, Allison James, Gerison Lansdown, Ann Oakley, Ginny Morrow, Helen Penn, Alan Prout, Jens Qvortrup, Helen Turner, Helga Zeiher.

I am deeply indebted to colleagues who collaborated with me on the studies referred to in this book: Gill Bendelow, Sandy Barker, Pamela Storey, Marijke Veltman, Peter Kelley, Suzanne Hood, Helen Turner.

Many people gave me time, thoughts and fun during 'fieldwork': children, school staff and parents. The work could not have been done without them!

The Economic and Social Research Council granted me a Research Fellowship (ref. No. R000 27 1056), specifically to write this book. I am very grateful to the ESRC for giving me this time.

1 | Introduction

The only route forward for sociological investigation if it is to achieve any detachment from the particular interests and values of the society in which the sociologist is working is to assume the equal moral worth of the inputs of all the workers involved, however they may rank each other and whatever deference or superiority they may exhibit.

(Stacey and Davies 1983: 16)

This book is an attempt to work towards a sociology for childhood. It works towards including children and childhood within sociological thinking: children as participant agents in social relations, and childhood as a social group fundamentally implicated in social relational processes. This is a less unfamiliar enterprise than it would have been 15 years ago, but it is still difficult and necessarily tentative. Broadly I am following in the footsteps of those who worked to include women's work both at home and elsewhere in the division of labour, and thus to problematize the public/private divide; and to theorize women as a social group within the gendered relations of ruling. With childhood and adulthood, as with women and men, we are concerned with processes in relations between social positions. And, as gender emerged as key to understanding social relations between women and men, generation is emerging as key to understanding relations between childhood and adulthood. Further, alerted as we are to take account of gender in social relations, we will now have to take account of intersections of gender with generation.

This book uses data collected with a few of the UK's children – those I have worked with in London, in the 1990s, in order to think from their lives towards sociological understanding. Here again, I am following feminists in their perception (following Marx) that the underdog provides essential evidence of the workings of the social order – the degree of 'fit' between assumptions and prescriptions of the ruling social order and people's experiences and understandings. Just as women in relation to male-structured social institutions are 'valuable strangers' (Harding 1991: 124), so we can learn from children about gaps and misfits between their experiences and their positioning in the social order, taken for granted by adults.

The analysis of the social order, taking account of children's perspectives, is essentially political – it is in favour of the upgrading of childhood as social status, taking account of respect for children as moral agents, of their contributions to the social order and of their rights. But the book does not move towards specific prescriptions towards recognition of children's rights; rather I aim to contribute to rights agendas by demonstrating their agency, and by theorizing their contributions. Thus I try to demonstrate that children have socially ascribed responsibilities and do fulfil them. As Knutsson (1997: 42) points out, children and childhood are 'embedded' in society and therefore in economy, government and culture. It is not that we should base the argument for children's rights on the fact that they carry responsibilities; it is that recognition of their responsibilities may help raise their social status, and thence provide an arena for serious consideration of their rights.

Studies of modern childhoods

My work over the last 10 years has taken place amidst a rapid expansion in the numbers of papers and books on the sociology of childhood, during which people have tried out various ways of theorizing or sociologizing childhood. I will come back to some of these in due course, but some of the most important – and ones that have influenced me – should be acknowledged at the outset: Jens Qvortrup, whose work has been seminal and who organized the 16-nation Childhood as a Social Phenomenon project (1985, 1991, 1994); Leena Alanen who has consistently produced thought-provoking theoretical work (1988, 1992, 2001); Chris Jenks who early on (1982) raised the problem – how may we think about 'the' child – in his book drawing together papers by key thinkers on the topic, and whose later book (1996) provides a thorough exploration of Parsons and Piaget, and of current dilemmas (especially around child protection); Allison James and Alan Prout, whose edited book of papers (1990, with a second edition in 1997) explored how sociological thinking on childhood would differ from psychological; James, Jenks and Prout (1998) who have drawn their forces together to reconsider models of childhood.

Since the mid-80s, a number of academic observers have identified factors that lead them to say modern childhood is a matter newly of great concern, and even in crisis. One argument is that the boundaries between childhood and adulthood are drawn ever more distinctly, as children's lives are separated out from those of adults (Qvortrup 1985); and age-patriarchy is ever more firmly enforced (Hood-Williams 1990). Zelizer (1985) analysed the removal of children from paid work, their devaluation as economic contributors and their status now as precious but burdensome. Wyness (2000: 1) argues that 'a recurring set of dominant ideas within political and academic domains . . . draws a generational boundary between adults and children, in the process restricting children to subordinate and protected social roles' and that this conception needs serious revision: we should accept that children are less reliant than before on adults and can take more responsibility for their own affairs (see also Scraton 1997). The notion of the child as threat in public spaces is a further cause for concern, and along with traffic danger and stranger danger, accounts for the exclusion of children from public places (Valentine 1996). And given children's alleged moral inferiority to adults, as apprentices within a scholarized childhood, children's rights become both a hot and a highly contested political issue (e.g. Scarre 1989a). However, another view is that childhood is disappearing in that young people's access to adult cultural worlds is blurring distinctions between childhood and adulthood (Postman 1983). The new media are giving children expertise in manipulating media and knowledge; and their access to sex and drugs is further blurring boundaries, making children stressed and rushing them too fast through what should be a carefree and innocent period of life (for review see Buckingham 2000: Chapter 2). One way and another, commentators argue: 'Indisputably, over the last two, or at most three, decades childhood has moved to the forefront of personal, political and academic agendas' (James *et al.* 1998: 5).

Such arguments, deriving from statistics, historical analysis and observation of social trends constitute provocative ways in to thinking about childhood. In Leena Alanen's terms (1998), these arguments are produced from the standpoint of 'looking down', from the large-scale, and from the adult point of view. They provide broad views across the terrain which help us think – about theory, rights, policy. However, it can be argued that, as with hooliganism (Pearson 1983), one can find intense concern or crisis about childhood in any period. Harry Hendrick's review (1997) of British constructions of childhood since 1800 points us to variations since then within longstanding concern about the character of childhood. It is well documented that academics and policymakers in western countries have been worried about childhood for at least a century and a half, since the state began to assume some responsibility for how and where children spent their time (at work in factories or as pupils in schools). State responsibility for children led swiftly to state worry about the division of labour – whether parents, and specifically mothers, and more specifically working-class mothers, took enough responsibility for children. Concern, from the mid-nineteenth century onwards, has focused on, for instance, infant mortality, child health, child labour, street children, the education of the lower classes, maternal neglect and ignorance, children as victims and as threats (e.g. Hurt 1979; Davin 1990; Cunningham 1991; Hendrick 1994). Indeed according to these commentators, one motive for corralling children into schools was to reduce their dangerous presence on the streets. Moral panics and arguments about divisions of responsibility – between parents and the state – have been around a long time.

This book aims to contribute to debates about childhood. It will include some looking down sections, but it will also look up from childhood, and, as recommended by Mills (1967), it aims to move productively between these two stances. I use children's own accounts to analyse their social status and social condition. Broadly, the philosophy and method underpinning how the book is written derive from feminism; just as Sandra Harding (1991) argued for 'thinking from women's lives', in order to construct knowledge, so here I am trying to think from children's lives, as recounted by them. And, as the book title suggests, the aim is to work towards a sociology for childhood – to help improve the social and political status of childhood. As Dorothy Smith put it, again in discussing work for women, the sociological aim: 'is not to explain people's behaviour, but to be able to explain to them/ourselves the socially organised powers in which their/our lives are embedded and to which their/our activities contribute' (1999: 8). Smith argues that through studying some women's lives we understand all women's lives better. The analogy is not direct for the study of children's lives, but perhaps we can say, if we put the study of children and childhood alongside the study of women's lives, we/women and children will begin to understand better our place in the socially organized power structures – the relations of ruling.

In this book I am using small samples from one corner of the world. As I have suggested, the aim is to use the data in order to theorize about childhood. I have not attempted to consider the world's children. This is because all I could do there would be to review the literature, and because I think this is not relevant to the theoretical enterprise of this book. What has seemed important is to think from the lives and accounts of a few children whom I got to know. I hope that my analysis of concepts and themes which emerge in the toing and froing between private troubles and public issues will be useful to others in thinking about how far the discussion resonates with childhoods they know of.

Approaches to studying childhood

In this book I bear in mind the point that history and sociology have much the same aims; they study two main issues: how did this thing (whatever the topic is) come about? and what is it or how is it best described? (Abrams 1982: 301). I accept the view of most key sociological thinkers (see review in Abrams 1982) that any attempt to consider a topic sociologically must take account of factors that have impinged over time – and this approach will form part of my consideration of childhood in this book. We have to ask, how has it come about that childhood is understood in the ways it is, in this society and at this time? I think that study of this question is helped by comparison; in Chapter 8 I compare some present-day English childhoods, with some present-day Finnish childhoods – for their histories and therefore their presents differ dramatically.

I am much encouraged in starting to write this book by the points made by Derek Layder (1998a, especially Chapter 6) where he argues that doing social research is a process of developing theory in the light of data. He calls this 'adaptive theory'.

> Adaptive theory both shapes and is shaped by the empirical data that emerges from research. It allows the dual influence of extant theory (theoretical models) as well as those that unfold from (and are enfolded in) the research. Adaptive theorising is an ever-present feature of the research process.
>
> (Layder 1998a: 133)

Thus at the start of a research project, one may hold some theoretical views, or have some theoretical concerns or hunches that one wants to test against data, in order to consider what may best fit or explain the data to be collected. During the course of data collection, analysis and 'writing up', one may modify those theories, through reading and discussion and study of the data. These modifications may provide new angles on an existing theory, new subsets within theory. One may also develop new theories, or call on other theories which seem to be relevant to the topic in hand.

Layder's (1994, 1997, 1998a, 1998b) understanding of what it is one does in social research and what it is appropriate to do, is a fitting prescription for our times. Like other commentators (e.g. Craib 1992; Delanty 1997), he notes the bewildering variety of sociological theories currently on offer, and the difficulties of defining a role for social theorists in relation to society; he concludes that 'there is no one theory or school of theory that has so far been able to adequately chart the connections between macro and micro phenomena in a comprehensive manner' (1994: 222). He argues that the best one can do is to work with 'disciplined eclecticism'; to take a multiperspectival approach harnessed to a programme of empirical research, such that theory and empirical evidence feed off each other (Layder 1994: 222). Thus Layder is responding to a social world where theories proliferate, and where the idea that one may understand small-scale data in the context of any one set of understandings of the whole society has lost currency.

It is interesting to compare his approach with Mills' (1967), which was first published in 1959. He famously proposed that one must look back and forth between the empirical and the theoretical, and between 'private troubles' and 'public issues' (Chapter 1). He similarly argued for the social theorist to regard his (*sic*) work as a process, wherein he works over a long period through a problem or set of problems, juxtaposing empirical data with reflection on how experience relates to larger issues.[1] And, notably, he did a hatchet job both on grand theorists, who pontificate from their ivory towers without stepping down into the dust of the arena (Chapter 2) and on mindless empiricists (Chapter 3). Mills had a grand vision of the social scientist's task and abilities; his lifetime task is to study the structure of this particular society as a whole, where it stands in human history, and what varieties of men and women now prevail in this society in this period (Chapter 1). Writing at a time when positivism was orthodoxy in American sociology, he argued strongly that sociology had a social role in criticizing power. The sociologist, and 'he' is 'usually a professor' (Mills 1967: 186), should use his working life in order to carry out this large and daunting task, but so is Layder a professor, and his goals are more modest – in keeping with the range and variety of current sociological theory.

Those of us who work as contract researchers (a gendered occupation) are less favourably positioned than Mills. As I said, the main material I am using derives from funded projects I carried out in the 1990s on childhood, over a period when social scientists were thinking about theory and empirical data and trying to map out a new territory – that of the sociology of childhood. Of course, as anyone familiar with contract research will recognize, the precise projects one carries out are dependent on funders' willingness to fund them. In my case, 28 per cent of my proposals to the main funding body for social science research were funded. However, the central problems I was pursuing were present in all the studies I aimed to do and did do, and in this sense they constitute a programme of work.[2]

Organization of the book

This book uses data from a range of studies, including four of mine, and explorations into theoretical concerns in order to work towards a sociology of and for childhood. How to organize material is an everpresent issue when writing up research. The natural history approach has some advantages – it may present events, thoughts, influences and discussions as they occurred, and so explain links and processes. But there are dangers in this approach: hindsight shapes the history; the storytelling may be chaotic, since components of the research process do not occur discretely or in ordered sequence during the work (Hammersley and Atkinson 1983: 215–17). However, Chapter 2 does adopt a storytelling approach in order to explain how my studies in the 1970s and 1980s led me to some basic ideas that are important in this book: that children are a minority social group; and that feminism was important – theoretically and in its methods. I try to show too how I made linkages between the empirical and theoretical: looking up from children's accounts to feminist analyses of women's people work and intermediate domain work.

Chapter 3 is based on reading done in preparation for the fourth study and later on in preparation towards this book. It introduces key themes – that childhood must be understood as a relational category, and therefore that generation (analogous to gender in feminist work) is a key concept for the study of childhood. Mannheim's work is useful here. The chapter points up the importance of including a historical dimension in sociological research, and pays tribute to the usefulness of critical realism as theoretical underpinning for studying relational processes.

Chapters 4, 5, 6 and 7 draw considerably on young people's accounts and the organization of the chapters is guided by the points they emphasize.[3] The young people in my London studies spend most of their days at home and at school, with brief forays into spaces in between. They describe family relations as central to their happiness and identities (Chapter 4), and school as the other main setting of their days (Chapter 5); consideration of the scholarization thesis leads to discussion of children as workers and how they understand this idea. A central theme that emerges from their talk across these two settings is the contested character of their moral agency and moral status, and so I give this major theme a chapter on its own (Chapter 6).

The next two chapters explore further ways of understanding childhood as a social phenomenon. In Chapter 7, I draw on young people's accounts of childhood in order to consider possibilities for the idea of a child standpoint; where through contextualizing their accounts in the social conditions of their lives one may reach a distinctive child view on their social status. Chapter 8 approaches the task of accounting for present-day childhoods through a comparison: 9-year-olds in a Finnish town live different lives from those in my London studies, and consideration of the history of childhoods as understood in the two countries may throw some light on these differences.

Finally, Chapter 9 takes up and reviews the themes of the book. The chapter considers the contribution of Mannheim to our understanding of generational processes and to the notion of a cohort of children as constituting a generation. I discuss the proposition outlined in this chapter: that childhood is in crisis, and consider possibilities for advancing children's rights. I take up the issue of relations between feminism and childhood studies, and suggest ways of working towards a sociology for childhood which takes account of both gender and generation. Key themes in developing a sociology for childhood – they run through the book (and are derived from feminism) – are: children in the division of labour, children as agents in the intermediate domain, and the idea of a child standpoint.

Overall, I take the view that childhood as a social position or category is a permanent component of the social order. In sociology we have to try to include childhood in, rather than exclude it from, consideration of how the social order works. Otherwise that consideration will be partial. In this book I have explored childhood as contributory to the social order, through childhood work – in schools and in person work – and through activities in the intermediate domain. I argue that those inhabiting childhood have a particular take or viewpoint on their status in relation to adult status, and that study of how their experiences may be accounted for by societal factors amounts to arguing that a child standpoint (analogous to a women's standpoint) is important for contributing to a proper account of the social order.

2 | Studying childhood

Introduction

There are various ways of approaching the study of childhood as a social phenomenon. One way is to review the literature, draw out from it the principal themes that seem to be part of the current *Zeitgeist*, and either leave it at that, or emphasize those that take one's fancy. Another way is to take the example of one empirical project and by looking back and forth between data and theory to construct a set of understandings of childhood. There is a difference of purpose between those who stand back from the fray and describe what is happening in research, and those for whom the aim is to present a specific point of view. There are also issues to be confronted as to whether one is interested in the development of theory, for the sake of better understanding, or whether one wishes to take things a step further and consider what those theories suggest for policy.

At present, the development of theory about childhood is an important sociological task. It is part of the task to relate private troubles to public issues within a theoretical framework. I regard children as a minority social group, whose wrongs need righting, in particular in the UK, and I do think that a clear theoretically informed understanding of the social status of childhood in relation to adulthood is an essential key to working towards righting those wrongs. This book is therefore offered as an attempt to provide a particular set of theoretical understandings of childhood, and it will explore implications of these for policy. But it is not a tract which in itself aims to change childhoods. I think the researcher's job is to help explain how things are, but it is not to presume to build on those (probably partial or transitory) explanations as a basis for entering the arena of political activism. Nor am I suggesting that my account of childhood has claims for important status, only that these are my attempts to present and analyse data and move towards a sociology for childhood.

In this chapter, I explain how and why I have focused on the areas of knowledge that have influenced my current ideas about childhood. This is offered not as justification but as explanation of the bases for these ideas. Anything we experience and learn from changes us, on both personal and professional levels; every time one's view of the world shifts, one begins to see things one has not seen before, or to see them differently (Craib 1992: 250). I embark on this task through a retrospective journey through the late 1970s onwards and in particular through reconsideration of four studies I carried out from 1990 to 1999. This retrospective and storytelling task entails problems. How do you remember what were the concerns at the time, and how they have developed? I have memories, and publications from these studies. I also have fieldnotes and the data – and have continued to read this material and think about it. But choice will be selective, and the very act of writing paragraphs and ordering them gives a new shape and direction to the topics.

Looking back and looking forward

Women's work, children's work?

During the 1970s and 1980s I worked on studies on mothers' care of their pre-school children and on the services they used and wished for (Mayall and Petrie 1983; Mayall 1986; Mayall and Foster 1989). During these studies I discussed with mothers (and a few fathers where available): childcare at home, their use of health services and daycare, and their relationships with providers of these services.[1] How life worked out for mothers was an important topic for study, and how mothers' happiness varied with their children's happiness emerged as a critical feature in their discourse. This was an era of important developments in feminist studies, so-called second-wave feminism. I was much influenced at this time by the work of Margaret Stacey, who had gathered together a team at Warwick University to consider *the division of labour* in child health-care between the various participants – the paid and the unpaid. Stacey and Davies' final report (1983) on their programme of studies became a sort of bible for me, and I made a memorable visit to Meg Stacey's house to read (and borrow and photocopy) working papers from their studies. They problematized the traditional ('malestream') division of the social order into the public and the private, a division which assumed that 'work' was a feature of the public domain, whilst activity in the private domain was not work – it was natural. Stacey and her team argued that '*people work*' (working on and for people) is carried out by women at home and by people working as, for instance, health visitors and social workers.[2] They further developed the important insight she had earlier pointed to: that the notion of the 'consumer' of health services is a 'sociological misconception' (1976); people should not be understood as passive objects of service-providers' work; they should be seen as workers. In an important paper on the division of labour, Stacey sets out this point in detail (1981: 186), and she notes that study of the division of labour must take account of children, 'for children work and are worked on' (1981: 187). At the time, this was a near-revolutionary concept, since children were currently understood as the objects of adult work and concern, within the general sociological view (based on psychological concepts) that childhood was a period of adult–child socialization, preparatory to participation as an adult in social life.

The idea that what women do at home should be counted as work led on to the Warwick proposition that important negotiations between paid and unpaid women take place in an *intermediate domain*, an arena where state/public interests and family/private interests intersect. The interventions of the preventive child health services, staffed by women in low status jobs (health visitors, clinical medical officers), could be seen as intrusions into 'the family' but they were mediated by the interactions between these paid women staff and mothers, both of whom work for and with children. Thus the idea of the intermediate domain allows for consideration of how *the gendered relations of ruling* (Smith 1988) operate within modern welfare societies, where power rests with high status male professionals, but where an ambiguous zone has been created 'where the concepts and values of the public domain mingled and conflicted with the values of the domestic domain' (Stacey and Davies 1983: 13). I later took up the notion of gender issues in relation to the intermediate domain by discussing the distinctive relationships child health services staff developed with mothers, as compared to those with fathers (Mayall 1993).

The notion of the intermediate domain resonated with data from our London studies of mothers' contacts with health and pre-school services. Mothers were powerless to change the structures that defined and controlled services, but they worked within these to negotiate the status of their knowledge and to construct adequate relationships – on behalf of their children – with health staff, and with childminders, nursery nurses and nursery teachers. If children could be regarded as agents within these services, people who participated in the structuring of their own days, as workers, rather than as objects of the services, then did this change one's understanding of the intermediate domain? This became a topic for consideration when I designed the first of four studies focusing on children's own activity (the Greenstreet Study, p. 14, this volume).

The period of the Warwick studies was also that of an advancing tide of conservatism, leading to the Conservative parliamentary victory in 1979 and 18 years of rule. This period, among other things, was characterized by glorification of the family, by privatization and brash capitalism and the rolling back of the welfare state – at least in rhetoric if not much in practice (Pilcher and Wagg 1996). It was a very difficult period for women struggling to assert their rights and working towards better social status. It was also a period when feminist publications from the early 1970s onwards were reaching the consciousness of those of us who, not active in the women's movement, were nevertheless working to understand, through empirical research, the lives of women and their children. Whilst some feminists struggled to emancipate themselves (at least theoretically) from the family (and its children), arguing that the family was a critical site of women's oppression and that physical motherhood did not necessarily imply social motherhood (e.g. Mitchell 1971; Oakley 1972; Rowbotham 1973; Barrett and McIntosh 1982), some feminists proposed that intersections between the sociopolitical position of women and children had to be explored.

Thus Dorothy Smith (1974, 1988), from a Marxist–feminist perspective, argued that women, themselves oppressed, work towards the maintenance of the social order by oppressing their children. From a slightly different angle, Shulamith Firestone (1971: Ch. 4) argued that it was the common oppression of women and children that tied them together; her solution was encapsulated in the chapter title: Down with childhood! But, the general trend in feminism grew from women's perception of the pressing need to problematize women's sociopolitical position; and this drive took precedence in most feminists' work over a coordinated attempt to rethink womanhood in intersections with childhood. They were concerned essentially with adult gender relations. For me, the problematics of childhood these authors briefly raised suggested that in the study of childhood consideration of the division of labour must be central. What difference would it make to sociological theory if we took account of children's participation? Did it make sense to conceptualize children as people workers, who contributed to their own health-care, and to social relations within the health-maintenance practices of the home? Did children regard themselves as oppressed by mothers? And even if they did not, was it relevant for the onlooker to suggest that they were? Should the concept of the intermediate domain – where women negotiate for children's welfare – be enlarged to take account of children as health-care actors?

The status of children and childhood

So by the middle of the 1980s, important influences were the concepts developed within feminism: debates on the division of labour, the idea that people are not 'patients' but health-care workers, the idea that women negotiate the status of their knowledge and practice in an intermediate domain in order to reach a reasonable deal within male-dominated structures. I was increasingly interested in where children were socially and politically positioned within these contexts, and how far they could be regarded as contributors – to the division of labour, to health-care work and to negotiations between women, to negotiating on their own behalf for a reasonable deal.

I was alerted as a mother to thinking about childhood, but also because, as a researcher, I saw at first-hand, on estates, in homes, on streets, at nurseries and minders, that children got a raw deal at the hands of policy-makers. In the 1970s and 1980s, when other European countries were providing universalist high quality state-run nurseries, British pre-school children were (and still are) the victims of a ramshackle patchwork of poor services. Indeed, as we bitterly noted (Hughes *et al.* 1980: Ch. 5), they could not be called services, but rather an ad hoc system which operated certainly not in the interests of children, nor even of the people who ran them, and certainly not for 'working' mothers, who struggled to finance the household in the face of inaccessible, insecure and unaccountable 'provision'. And since child poverty was (and still is) a running sore in the UK, the conditions in which many children lived (and still live) their lives at home and in the neighbourhood were appalling (Rahman *et al.* 2000; Hood 2001).

It was therefore very important to try to understand why children's social status was so low, by gaining access to the knowledge that was being developed in the wider world beyond these shores. I think Jens Qvortrup's 1985 paper was the first I read on the sociology of childhood, in which he argued that the scholarization of children – as a consequence of industrialization – had shifted ideas about the value of children. Whereas they had been valued for their direct economic contribution to their family and to the labour market, now they were thought of as dependants being socialized; their school activity was regarded as preparatory. By contrast Qvortrup argued that we should think of children's school work as work, as economically valuable. He organized the 16-country programme Childhood as a Social Phenomenon (CSP) (1987–92); this focused on the legal, economic and social status of children in industrialized countries and on their daily activities, as evidenced in large-scale data (Qvortrup 1991). Its work began to filter through the networks to researchers in the UK. As he explained in a paper published in 1990, the CSP's main proposition was 'that children are active and constructive members of society and that childhood is an integral part of society'. That paper appeared in James and Prout's seminal edited collection of papers (1990; 2nd edn. in 1997), in which they set out distinctions between psychological and sociological understandings of childhood and provided a set of papers which addressed key issues, among them: the history of ideas about childhood (Hendrick); the concept of children's needs (Woodhead); and the globalization of western concepts of childhood (Boyden).

Research studies on and with children

In 1990, a time when childhood research was not yet on the agenda of most funding bodies,[3] I was very fortunate that the Institute of Education under-wrote some of my salary, and this, together with a project grant from the enlightened Nuffield Foundation, allowed me to start off on what turned out to be a programme of childhood research.[4]

The Greenstreet Study (1990–2)
When planning the proposal for this project, I decided to aim for a study which would ask children themselves for their experiences of daily life. I remember thinking that it might be difficult to work with pre-schoolers (though nowadays researchers have successfully worked with 3- and 4-year-olds). So I planned to move slightly up the age-range and to focus on reception class children (4–6 years old) getting their first taste of school, as well as on older ones (9–10 years old), who had several years of school experience. The particular focus of this study was on children as health-care actors at home and at school.

This planned study was for me a first, in that it focused directly on children as the centre of research attention. I carried out the fieldwork in one primary school, over two terms, in 1990 and 1991. I collected data informally from the children, at school, in pairs and singly and groups, and also talked with most of the teaching and non-teaching staff. And I interviewed some of the mothers at home (with the children present and contributing if they wished).

The Greenstreet Study aimed to consider intersections between how children experience and act within the home and school, and how they are understood by adults in those settings. In brief, it showed that, whilst at home mothers understand their children by the age of 4 or 5 as competent health carers, under their mothers' care and control, at school teachers regarded children as lacking competence and maturity, and school required them to subjugate their bodily selves to the school's regime and official remits. This was more difficult for the younger than for the older children, who had learned to manage and to some extent negotiate the social order. In terms of power relations, parental power was mediated by the desire to encourage children's control and autonomy; teachers' power was directed towards conformity. Children played little part in the intermediate domain negotiations between mothers and teachers, and this lack further served to diminish their social and political status at school.

The study provided a basis for further research funding applications, and the next successful application funded a study which followed on directly from it. By now I felt confident that data could be collected with children in their early school years, and that the themes within the notion of the division of labour could be pursued taking account of children's contributions. By putting children's health (maintenance, promotion and restoration) at school at the centre of the research, the study focused on intersections of education and health, and at a time when concern about the underfunding of schools was growing, it proved a fundable proposition.

The CHIPS Study (1993–5)
The study addressed the broad question: what is the status of children's health in primary schools? It consisted of a postal survey of a random sample of primary schools in England and Wales (620 schools). After initial analysis of this, we carried out case studies in six schools. The survey, addressed to headteachers, asked about staff–child ratios, the school's physical characteristics, health education policy, arrangements for maintaining and restoring children's health (meals, physical activity, provision of a sick room and trained staff), and input by other agencies including the school health service. In the case-study schools, chosen to reflect variety in size, age-range, geographical and socioeconomic location, the same topics were addressed, and our informants included children aged 6 and 10, teaching and non-teaching staff, parents, and school health service staff.

This study considered the division of labour at differing levels. It provided information on the input of various services into schools, and allowed for elucidation of the separation between health and education at ministerial, local authority, and school levels; it showed how responsibility for the care of children at school is divided up between staff (and differs between schools). It also pointed to splits in thinking about children, again at all levels. The physical and psychological and cognitive components of children belonged to different ministries and to different local services; within schools children and teachers balanced the bodily, emotional and cognitive as priorities in the school day, with the cognitive tending to predominate under teacher control.

Thus the study allowed for reflection on the social and political status of children and of childhood at primary school. Again, there are points to be made at different levels. Thus social assumptions allow for children's working conditions to be poor (by comparison with those legally enforced for adults), and our respondents judged the buildings, toilets, playgrounds and classroom space as poor in many cases. In local authority policy, children's health has low priority in school, judging by the absence of demarcated spaces to care for them, by the (generally rare) input of the school health service, and by cutbacks in other health-related services (for special needs, chronic conditions, and for referral to specialist care). Children have little opportunity for participation in decision-making about any aspect of their school experience. Their own understandings of links between the bodily, emotional and cognitive did not always meet with staff recognition. However, in the majority of their reports of illness and accident at school, they found that staff cared for them well (76 and 83 per cent respectively).

This study showed how children's experience is sited within the material and ideological 'school' as an institution established across time and in space. Thus education policies and traditions, established over many years, structured experience. For instance, the length of the school day, with its breaks and dinnertime, its assemblies (with a broadly religious component) require staff and children to reproduce social relations rooted in the past. Old school buildings, built with an eye to past education policies and services, continue to impact on this generation of children – who commented on the (un)suitability of the buildings and playspaces for their daily lives. Both staff, and to a lesser extent children, take part in modifying these social and physical structures to suit current demands.

The division of labour in schools is structured through the gender order. Primary schools are staffed very largely by women – as teachers, secretaries, dinner ladies; this gender dimension complements the traditional view of the primary school as a follow-on from the home, where the teacher is 'the mother made conscious' (Steedman 1988). These women work within the structures laid down by higher authority – the reified or objectified complex of social relations : the relations of ruling (Smith 1999: Ch. 5). These not only control the formal agenda, but assume that women's work will include a caring component. Thus, though employers of adults must ensure there are first-aiders (one for 50 staff), this provision is not in place for children. In our survey, there was wide variation; 13 per cent of schools had no one with any training (on minimal criteria). In practice, according to case-study children's accounts of recent accident and illness, they turned to teachers and non-teaching staff fairly equally for help. Women staff both control and care for the children, and some children's reports indicate that good child–adult relationships and satisfactory experiences at school are cemented by the women's caring work. This point acts as a commentary on Dorothy Smith's argument (1988) that women work oppressively on and with children in the service of the relations of ruling.[5] Children's own perspectives suggest that women's caring work at school can mitigate the harshest features of the institution's domination of children.

These two empirical research projects had allowed for consideration of the division of labour in childcare, including the contribution of children themselves. It was clear that the home constituted a distinctive health-care environment compared to the school; at home children's drive towards self-care was valued, since mothers understood their children as competent people who seek independence; at school, staff did not recognize children's competence and instead emphasized their immaturity; staff's overriding concern was with implementing the formal school agendas. With hindsight, the study of childhood experience at school shows intersections of gender and generation. Not only do women and children as social groups each find themselves defined and controlled in certain ways; they act in tension or collaboratively to humanize the environments in which they work.

Judging by the publications arising from these two studies, I was mainly concerned at the time with the social status of children and of childhood, and in thinking about children's opportunities for modifying the social settings within which they lived. Childhood emerged as a social status where people's experience is firmly shaped by structures over which they have little influence. This position made me start to look for theory that recognized distinctions between agency and structure, rather than theory which – in any of the variants – tended to fuse the two (see pp. 32–5). Such fusions seemed to me both to de-emphasize power relations, and to give precedence to agency over structure; in both respects such fusion seemed not to fit with how childhood is lived.

The Risk Study (1995–6)

This was an exploratory study of child–parent relationships pinned on the topic: how do children and parents understand the home – is it a risky environment for children? The aim was to explore people's understandings of intersections of home and locality, home and politics, home and school/education. Fieldwork for this qualitative study took place in a socially and ethnically mixed neighbourhood in inner London; it focused on children aged 3, 9 and 12 years and their parents and included one-off interviews in 45 households and some discussions with children at school.

We explored Ulrich Beck's (1992) thesis that nowadays we live in a 'risk society', developed through the global production of risks, many of them invisible and unpredictable, and through the restructuring of advanced societies, which has freed people from social class and career determined by parental position, and has led to the individualization of careers; life-courses have become less certain, more reflexive, more a matter of individual choice and agency. Beck argues that in some 'advanced' societies a socioeconomic order structured through inequalities in wealth distribution has been replaced by a social order characterized by the distribution of risk, and that 'the type, pattern and media for the distribution of risks differ systematically from those of the distribution of wealth' (1992: 35). The child is not an agent in Beck's account, but he identifies the value of children; in a world of transient unreliable relationships, the child is 'the source of the last remaining, irrevocable, unexchangeable primary relationship. Partners come and go. The child stays' (1992: 118). We drew on Beck's theories, first, to explore whether our sample parents lent support to his account of the risk society and his individualization thesis. Did they understand social, environmental and economic contexts as risky and hostile, or as supportive and trustworthy? Did they think biographies structured by social class and gender were being replaced by increasingly individualized biographies? Were parents having to make more choices about work, where to live and children's education, and if so how were risk-related ideas implicated in the decision-making process?

But second, since the children might be regarded (by us, by parents, by themselves) as a new generation, we wanted to explore whether their own lives and choices were determined by their parents' biographies. If children are regarded as a social group, located in a specific time and social space, then perhaps as a group they might be differentially affected by factors affecting parents. So for example transport policies, the marketized education system, discourses on children's rights might have specific effects on decision-making in children's lives.

According to our end-of-project report, the study suggested strongly that these children and parents live in a society where wide differences between social groups in financial and cultural terms meant that parents vary in what they can 'give' their children. For instance, well-to-do parents saw the home as a place of safety from risk, but home presented dangers for poorer parents (poverty, poor housing, illness). As ever, poorer parents, and those with less knowledge of how to play the system (social capital in Bourdieu's (1986) terms) felt unable to choose and access 'good' schools.

This study was centrally concerned with intergenerational relationships, with a particular focus on how childhood was understood and experienced by children, and how parental memories of childhood related to their parenting of their children. It explored intersections between generation and gender. But while parents' accounts suggest they did differ in their behaviour to daughters and sons in respect of the dangers of the outside world, children themselves regarded age, parity and status (as primary versus secondary schoolchildren) as more important factors determining their daily experience.

When we looked at the 'risk issues' from the point of view of the children, we concluded that children aged 9 and 12 regarded their negotiating power as severely limited by their subordinate position in child–parent relations, by their dependency on parents and by lack of knowledge. Their subordination included lack of control over both minds and bodies, both of which parents regarded as legitimate spheres for intervention. Their dependency was social as well as economic, and whilst they welcomed parental control and protection aimed at their physical safety, they were more resistant to socialization agendas which prioritized their future over their present.

This exploratory study provided tantalizing and fascinating data, but we failed to get funding for a more detailed study of them. However, a bit later on I did get funding for a detailed study of children's own understanding of childhood.

The Childhood Study (1997–9)

The central aim here, as the proposal stated, 'was to study how children's childhoods are experienced, understood and structured by them and by the adults and children with whom they have important relationships'. The study would (like an earlier Nordic study, see Alanen 1992) consider issues of gender and of integration and autonomy – how children's independence, personal and social identities are negotiated within the home and in wider socioeconomic contexts. It was to be a small-scale detailed study, including children living in a range of family types, and focusing on children near the top of primary school (Year 5, aged 9–10) and established in secondary school (Year 8, aged 12–13). In choosing two ages of childhood associated with the status of 'primary school child' and 'secondary school student' I would be able to discuss with children intersections of ideas about childhood with their status now and in the past.

In practice, the study included 139 children, and data were collected with them in pairs, individually and in groups. Initial discussions were on their concepts of childhood and parenthood; later on I asked them to describe and reflect on their experiences of daily life. The central focus was the study of children's relationships with adults and other children and the aim was to consider children's participation in constructing and maintaining relationships, including those with non-resident relatives (notably fathers and grandparents). It was concerned with how these relationships are negotiated in the context of modern London childhoods, where it is commonplace for parents' own relationships to change, for important people to move out and move in, and where parental work patterns offer challenges to adults' and children's ideas about how childhood should be lived.

The findings from this study are discussed in succeeding chapters, with references to relevant data from the three earlier studies, and in relation to the development of theory on childhood. However, in connection with the history given in this chapter, I flag up some of the points that emerged. Just as women experience disjunction (or a fault line) between how they experience their daily lives and how they think they are supposed to experience them, so children find a gap between ideas current in their environment about childhood and their actual experience. So-called 'family breakdown' and parental hours of work make demands on children outside normative notions of childhood. A topic of burning concern to children is their moral status; their experience of low moral status runs contrary to their insistence on their rights, especially their participation rights – and, from the observer's point of view, to the evidence they provide of their moral competence. The data also provide food for thought on children's participation in the division of labour, both at home and at school.

Learning to study childhood

Childhood as minority social status

My studies to this point had lent considerable support to the view that children are best regarded as a minority social group. In the first place, study of child–adult relations showed that childhood is understood by both adults and children as a time of dependency and subordination – among other things. Second, the notion that children need socializing is strong both among parents and in particular among teachers; children too voice the opinion that it is parents' responsibility to teach children morality (see also Montandon 2001). Third, the home and the school – the principal physical sites of modern London childhoods – are organized around the power of the adults to determine the character of children's experience.

Social setting emerged as a crucial determinant of children's experience. The home and the school offer, enable and enforce distinctive types of childhood, through the ideologies adults hold about childhood, through adults' own agendas, through current ideas about 'the home', 'the family' and 'the school'. As the CHIPS Study explored, the history of educational policy, congealed into buildings and outside space still used today, provides material bases for structuring children's experience. The history of London housing with its class divisions – spacious Victorian homes for some and cramped council flats for others, ensures distinctive lives at home for children and parents.

The 'scholarization' of childhood is such a visible feature of modern western childhoods that it may escape notice. But the fact that children are required for many years to spend a considerable portion of their time at school – and increasingly also to bring schoolwork home – has implications for how childhood is understood. Childhood as apprenticeship, as preparation, as separate from the economic mainstream of adult activity is an important component of modern UK ideas about childhood. In the eyes of some adults, modern childhood is less a time of freedom and exploration and more and more restricted; parents think they must compensate for this loss by providing organized leisure activities for their children. Even between 1990 and 1998, the period during which I listened to children talking about their lives, scholarization has widened and deepened its hold on London children. I think that the sheer amount of child activity demanded by schools nowadays may push adults towards rethinking how to describe what children do at and for school. What they do looks more and more like work. And this raises the question of how far it is appropriate to understand children as contributors to the division of labour.

These studies, in focusing on children's own accounts, raise issues about children's agency. It is clear enough, without carrying out formal research studies, that children are social actors; that is, they take part in family relationships from the word go; they express their wishes, demonstrate strong attachments, jealousy and delight, seek justice. But the research attempt to put children into sociology raises the issue whether they may be regarded as agents. Of course, the etymological root of 'agent' and 'actor' is the same Latin verb (*ago, agere, egi, actum*), but in usage the meanings of the two words have diverged somewhat. A social *actor* does something, perhaps something arising from a subjective wish. The term *agent* suggests a further dimension: negotiation with others, with the effect that the interaction makes a difference – to a relationship or to a decision, to the workings of a set of social assumptions or constraints.

Childhood agency has to be understood within the parameters of childhood's minority status. People who inhabit childhood differ from adults in that childhood is understood as a period when people require protection, since they know less, have less maturity and less strength, compared to older people; protection implies also provision; and it implies unequal power relationships. As commonly understood, childhood is a period of growing towards adulthood (for discussion of being and becoming in the life-course, see Lee 2001). So children's agency is influenced by this complex of understandings. In substantiating the proposition that children inhabit a minority social group, these studies draw attention to children's strongly expressed feeling for justice and equal shares, for participation in decision-making. Children talk in terms of the denial of their rights, even though few use the formal language of rights. This is particularly evident when they talk about their lives at school; they see themselves as a group vis-à-vis the adult group, and as a group whose rights are both neglected and rejected.

Finally, study of children's lives, as they and parents and teachers note, is essentially the study of child–adult relations. This leads on to the point that it is the study of relations between sets, or cohorts, of people growing up at differing times, exposed to differing sociopolitical processes. Parents in the Risk Study overtly contrasted their own childhoods with those of their children, whom they regarded as subjected to different sets of opportunities and constraints, compared to themselves when children. Teachers in the 1990s told me they found their work nowadays uncomfortable, because they belonged to a generation educated in child-centred educational principles, but were required to implement a curriculum based on a set of ideologies that ran counter to these.

Childhood sociologies

Anyone studying children must be grateful for the careful and revelatory work of psychologists. I pay tribute to some in this book. But I want here to point briefly to distinctiveness between psychological and sociological concerns. Studies of childhood in sociology and in developmental psychology have in some important respects become more similar since about the mid-1980s. Developmental psychology has become less universalist and more contextualized; it understands children as persons who contribute to their own learning, notably through interactions with other people (Rogoff 1990; Cole 1996; Woodhead 1997). Social psychological research has drawn attention to the critical importance of local ideologies of childhood and of intersections between child–adult relations and structures of the social order (Kagitcibasi 1996). Researchers have moved out of the laboratory to study real life situations, at home and in institutional settings (Woodhead *et al.* 1998), including children's own accounts of their lives. There are thus parallels with the work of some sociologists studying childhood.

However, at this point we have to take account of the more recent and con-current development of three main kinds of sociology taking children as their focus (Alanen 2001: 12–14). The first and most common may be called the *sociology of children*. Here the focus is on the child as agent, as participatory in constructing knowledge and daily experience; an important issue is children's own views on their daily experience, and these may be sought in order to construct an account of childhood. The intersections of children's experiences with the social worlds they inhabit, and notably their relations with other children and with adults, are a fundamental concern. Thus these 'sociological' explorations have similarities to recent psychological ones.

But long-established theoretical traditions continue to ensure that the dominant, and highly influential, concerns of developmental psychology continue to be distinctive.[6] Developmental psychology remains future-oriented; it wants to know how small people become big people. It concerns itself with difference, with factors that lead to good and bad outcomes. Its focus is commonly on the individual, and on local interactions. This means it has been and is generally now apolitical.

By contrast the sociology of children, as it has developed in more recent years, is inherently interested in the present tense of childhood – the character of people's experience now. And second, though it too is concerned with difference, most importantly it studies commonality – what binds children together as social group and distinguishes them from adults. Third, it is concerned with children as a social group, especially with children's relations with adults in their daily lives. These concerns imply that the sociological vision studies power relations and is fundamentally political. Thus the sociology of children has been important in documenting children's lives, recording and discussing their own expressed experiences and raising concerns about the character and quality of their childhoods.

A second strand in the development of sociological work on childhood has taken place in the wake of postmodern visions and methodologies. This *deconstructive sociology of childhood* draws attention to varying discourses about children and childhood (cf. Jenks 1996); it seeks to show how such discourses provide the spaces and times for people to enact childhoods as locally defined. As Jenks argues (1996: 13), 'We need to look at the reasons for the child, and the generative grounds of the image and the archetypes in our language.' He makes a powerful case for the construction of specific western childhoods in the twentieth century by two key figures: Talcott Parsons and Jean Piaget. The twin towers of sociology and psychology provide the interlocked and complementary framework for commonplace notions of childhood.

The third strand in sociological work on childhood may be called a *structural sociology of childhood*. Here we are concerned with childhood as a permanent social category in society. Its members change, but childhood, in its relations with the other major social group – adulthood (from which it is defined as different) – continues as an essential component of a social order where the general understanding is that childhood is a first and separate condition of the lifespan whose characteristics are different from the later ones. Much of the major work in this strand has been done through large-scale work (Qvortrup *et al.* 1994), where such major movements as industrialization, urbanization, scholarization have been analysed in relation to distributive justice, concepts of work, and the character of children's actual everyday lives.

The essentially relational structure of childhood in this third vision provides the basis for a generational approach to childhood, which will be an important feature of this book (see Chapter 3). Essentially, we are concerned with two interrelated issues: first, childhood as constituted in particular ways as a distinctive generational position – by contrast with adulthood; that is, we shall be studying 'generationing' processes (analogous to gendering processes), notably those set in train by earlier generations of adults, through which childhoods come to have certain characteristics. Second, we shall be interested in Mannheim's examination (within cultural theory) of how historical generations are formed. Bringing together these two strands is an important challenge, for one way to understand the historical particularity of present childhoods is through studying child–adult relationships mediated by adult – and child – biographies.

Feminism

During my journey through four studies, I have found feminist methods of work useful, by analogy, towards rethinking childhood. Feminists have provided a *critique* of traditional sociological concepts, showing how these have been devised from the point of view of men, and from positions of masculine power. They have re-analysed the division of labour to show that the concept of the social order as comprising public and private domains is a social construction, and to problematize the assumption that 'work' is only that which is done, for pay, in the public domain. They have filled in gaps in the sociological agenda by discussing issues previously neglected: housework, childbirth, child-rearing and sexual politics (e.g. Mitchell 1971; Oakley 1972). Jane Ribbens (1990) gave a feminist account of child-rearing; through identifying mothers' models of childhood as expressions of philosophical standpoints, she analyses mother–child relations as political expressions. In so doing she challenges the standard male distinction between an apolitical private sphere and a political public sphere.

These critiques opened the way to developing concepts that allow for analysing how the social order works, taking account of women. Women have shown how women's work underpins men's work; *the gender order* is integral to the relations of ruling (Smith 1999: 4–8). Similarly, we may argue, children's work underpins adults' work; the generational order is similarly a constituent part of the relations of ruling. Gendered structures find parallels in the *generational structures* that serve to organize childhoods: the adult control of knowledge about childhood; the exclusion from concepts of work of children's activity; the notion that children act within the private domain. Feminism teaches us to take account of gender in any consideration of social relations; in the case of childhood this means considering intersections of gender with generation; for instance we have to consider implications of the point that within homes and primary schools, it is mainly women who interact with children, but within social structures not of their own making.

Just as women were excluded from sociology – in the sense that the gender order was not recognized and problematized, so children and childhood have traditionally been excluded from sociological consideration, since – relying on psychological theory – sociologists regarded childhood as a preparatory, not participatory phase (e.g. Ryder 1965). Theoretically, then, the task is to consider how to make sociology fit for children.

Of course one can take the analogy only so far. The political enterprise of feminism differs in important ways from the enterprise of working for children (Oakley 1994). Feminists have fought for their own social group – women – though white middle-class women have been forced to recognize ethnic and social subdivisions (for review, see Segal 1995), whereas here we have adults fighting for a different social group – children. Yet children's own political activity and ways children can work with adults to raise the status of childhood are being developed.[7] There is also a set of issues around the (obvious) point that whilst men and women have never belonged to the other sex, we have all been children. Our adult views on children and childhood will be influenced by our own experience of childhood, but memories may falsify and distort. Our escape from childhood into adulthood may lead us to neglect children's interests, and the gendered division of labour in parenting has led feminists to resist 'being lumped together with children' (Firestone 1971: 101). In policy terms, it would take a revolution in parenting – so that fathers and mothers took equal shares – and a radical rethink of the division of people's time between paid work and home to provide a social order conducive to the serious consideration of children's rights.

Building on the critique of 'malestream' sociological concepts, feminists have taken up the point that to build an adequate sociology it is crucial to take account of *people's own experiential knowledge*, how they experience and understand the social world and the structures of knowledge that are not of their making. People's experience and their everyday activities are structured by the material conditions of their social positioning. These conditions are 'organized by relations external to the everyday world and beyond the power of individuals to control' (Smith 1988: 95). The task of the sociologist is to site women's experience and knowledge in the social and political contexts within which they live, and thus to work towards theorizing a *standpoint for women*: 'to explore how [experience] is shaped in the extended relations of larger social and political relations' (1988: 10). Smith argues that women experience a disjunction between their actual experience and how they are expected (by the dominant culture) to experience their daily lives.[8] Such disjunctions are identified too by children; there are differences between how they experience life and how, as a child, they are supposed to.

In later chapters, I shall discuss these issues, in particular focusing on child–adult relations in the family (Chapter 4) and at school (Chapter 5), children's moral status (Chapter 6) and on the usefulness of the idea of a child standpoint as a means of incorporating childhood into sociological understandings (Chapter 7). At this point, in summary, the implications of Dorothy Smith's valuable work for studying childhood seem to me to be three.

First, it is important to develop sociological thinking that is fundamentally relational. Just as gender emerged as a crucial concept for analysing relationships between the sexes, so generation is coming to be seen as key to understanding child–adult relationships. At all levels of analysis, one wants to maintain a focus on relational processes – how this thing has come about, and how it is working out now. We have to be concerned with individual relations, and relations between social groups. Second, we must take account of how children themselves experience and understand their lives and social relationships, and use this information to develop a child standpoint. And third, children's experiential knowledge is a vital ingredient in any effort towards the recognition of children's rights. In this book children's discourse will be considered in order to throw light on their understanding of their social position and how far their rights are respected. Just as feminism is essentially a political enterprise, so too must be childhood studies.

| Studying relational
processes

Introduction

This chapter will further explore ideas to be deployed in the book when discussing childhood as a structural component in society and the social condition of childhood as experienced by children. The attempt here is to work towards a relational sociology, that is to consider how it comes about that childhoods are constructed in various ways, through exploration of the designation of some people as children in contradistinction to others, designated as adults. In trying to construct a relational sociology, I draw on the suggestions made over the years by Jens Qvortrup (e.g. 1991, 1994) and by Leena Alanen (1992, 2000) that the most promising concept for considering childhood in its sociological relations to the social order is that of generation.

As outlined in Chapter 2, just as the concept *gender* was developed in order to analyse the ways in which women were defined in contradistinction to men, so the concept *generation* may serve comparable ends; we may reach an understanding of the character of childhood if we look at how it is defined in contradistinction to adulthood. But that is to present a static vision where definitions and social constructions look fixed. Women's work on gender quickly progressed from considering only the state of play – the social condition of women vis-à-vis men – towards exploring *gendering*, that is, exploring relational processes whereby definitions are both accomplished and changing. Similarly, we may propose the notion of *generationing*, through which we consider the relational processes whereby people come to be known as children, and whereby children and childhood acquire certain characteristics, linked to local contexts, and changing as the factors brought to bear change.

At this point, it becomes clear that a historical contribution is highly pertinent to considering processes in relations between adulthood and childhood. Whereas relations between, say, men and women or between ethnic groups can, for some purposes, be studied in terms of their relations to the social and temporal space they all live in as a cohort, that is as people born in roughly the same period of time, in the case of children this is not so. An important component of the differences ascribed to childhood compared to adulthood concerns their differing sitings in historical and social time. This difference and this relationality draws attention to intersections of past and present. In their relationships with adults, children find themselves faced with adult knowledge and experience derived from an earlier time. In turn, adults must face up to children's distinctive ways of understanding the social world, derived from their learning as members of a later cohort. It will therefore be important in this study to consider these intersections at many levels.

This chapter will weave together ideas drawn from historical sociology, critical realism and generational sociology in order to consider how these ideas help us to conceptualize childhood. The main points are brought together at the end of the chapter.

Childhood as relational process

I start here by setting out one kind of schema through which we may study children compared to adults, and childhood compared to adulthood. The sociological enterprise of considering relations between social groups or positions can be carried out at differing levels. The analysis in this book will shift back and forth between these levels.

Individual relations

In everyday living, people relate to each other as individuals; children and adults at home and school work through relationships and boundaries; they negotiate space, time and status. At individual levels, too, children learn the culture of their particular family. They participate with adults in the common enterprise of keeping the household going. Children's access to resources is shaped by the specific socioeconomic circumstances of their own family. The extent to which children's rights to protection, provision and participation are respected at home and school varies according to individual adult perspectives, resources and the local environment. In all these child–adult relations, gender provides a cross-cutting influence.

Within these individual interactions, too, history plays a part. People take knowledge drawn from their individual past in order to manage present challenges. For instance, a mother draws on her knowledge of her own past behaviour and of her child's character, behaviour and wishes in order to consider the best way of interacting with her child now, in the present. She may also draw on her own history as a child and adult; her goals for her child may draw on that history and may structure how she acts at any point in caring for and urging her child in specific directions (see Cole 1996: 183–5 on the concept of prolepsis). The family's particular customs and routines established over time provide a framework for children's days, and children interact with these customs and routines to reproduce and modify them.

Like adults, children make use of the knowledge they have from past experiences with parents in order to manage their interactions with them; they take account of character, moods, interests and dispositions. Children tell me that they can use this experiential knowledge at school when dealing with their primary school teacher since they get to know her well over the year, but when they get to secondary school they have much poorer knowledge about their teachers since there are many of them, children's time with each is short and fragmented, and teaching styles are more formal and distant.

Group relations at local levels

Here we are concerned with relations between the social positions of childhood and adulthood. At local levels these can be observed at their clearest in schools, where children identify themselves as a group which has to deal with the adult group – comprising, for example, teachers, classroom assistants and dinner ladies. Children commonly describe all these subgroups of adults as having authority over them, and as requiring children's compliance with the social order of the school. From children's points of view, adult authority over the group children predominates over gender issues. Siblings in family interactions also somewhat position themselves, for some purposes, as a group which faces up to parental authority; siblings make common cause to advance their interests as a group. For instance, they may throw their combined weight into an argument in favour of watching television or of playing out together, when their mother thinks they should be otherwise engaged.

It is worth noting here the common device in stories for children where the author positions a number of children, siblings or friends, outside the immediate authority of parents (who may be conveniently busy, dead, in gaol, or living elsewhere). Examples are many, but for instance: Enid Blyton's friendship group the Famous Five, and E. Nesbit's sibling groups – who have adventures on their own; Arthur Ransome's children who spend idyllic holidays on boats and islands away from their parents; J.K. Rowling's Harry Potter who leaves his nasty relatives to join the group of apprentice wizards at boarding school. The enduring popularity of such stories suggests that children identify strongly with children's agency as a social group, and enjoy stories which give power of independent action to children, in contradistinction to much of ordinary life where they are subject to adult authority.

Cohort effects – at individual levels

Relations between individual children and individual adults can be seen as affected by the fact that children belong to a different cohort from adults. (I understand 'cohort' here to mean people born at roughly the same point in historical and social time.) For instance, under-5s at the time of writing (summer 2001) were born into differing social conditions compared to their parents; small children now interact with computers, watch videos as well as live television, are more likely to attend nursery classes and will be introduced to literacy and numeracy earlier than their parents were. Children's specific types of competence derived from such experiences may be a factor in their relationships with their parents. By teaching their parents technological skills, they may raise their status in child–parent relations. The parents of these children grew up in a sociohistorical period when (they tell me) children had greater physical freedom than today's children; parents in my Risk Study drew on their memories of freedom to explore the neighbourhood when considering how to 'give' their children a childhood; they thought the outside world was risky; and debated how to compensate for protective strategies by escorting their children to safe environments (see Chapter 4).

Cohort effects at group levels

Here we are concerned with large-scale impacts of social policies on relations between cohorts of children and adults. Social policies that impact on childhood experience are constructed, whether by design or not, by cohorts of older people drawing on their own experience, and on their ideologies of childhood and adulthood and the correct relationships between childhood and adulthood. Thus housing, transport, welfare, education and health policies provide adult-designed structures for children's lives, structures that reflect earlier cohort identities, goals and ideologies. These policies, by and large, are designed without referring directly to the cohort children – what those called children now think is appropriate. The relationships between the adult group and the child group can be seen as shaped by the social policies constructed by the first group and experienced by both groups. Respect for children's participation rights is clearly important here – their rights to discuss the appropriateness of congealed social structures.

The social group children now also hold ideas that belong to their cohort. Children attending school through the 1990s have been exposed to profound changes in educational policies. They tell me that education is a matter of getting good grades, as a passport to a good job. They have absorbed an understanding of what education is which is in tune with the schooling they are getting; as a group, children's instrumental understanding contrasts with 'liberal' understandings among some parents.

Individuals, groups and cohorts

This is only one way of schematizing ways of approaching processes in child–adult relations. Interlinkages between levels could be set out differently – for instance, cohort could be subsumed under individual and group. My aim has been to outline differing levels at which one may approach the study of childhood. It is also to draw attention to how they come into play and relate to each other. Thus when we hear a child say to his mother, 'Let me go out and play on my bike!' we can consider the *individual relations* between child and mother, including the power relationship (for he has to ask permission); the mother's gendered understanding of her responsibility as a member of the *social group* mothers; her memories as a member of a *cohort* of children who rode bikes in the neighbourhood; the *social policies* that nowadays ensure the roads, and even the pavements, are not safe for children and *societal assumptions* about the division of state and parental responsibility for child welfare. The mother's thinking will take account of all these levels. The child will take account of his individual desire to ride freely outside, and of his intimate knowledge of his mother's character and past behaviour on this topic; at group level, he will argue that riding bikes is something children do, yet he will be aware that adults wish to protect and control, as well as care for children; his thinking and his interactions will also be modified by his knowledge that the outside world carries dangers.

Sociology and history

The discussion so far draws attention to the importance of past influences on the present. Sociology has to be concerned with the extent to which and ways in which the past influences or structures the present, how far agents reproduce, or transform what is already there. 'All sociology worthy of the name is "historical sociology". It is . . . an attempt to write "the present as history"' (Mills 1967: 146). Indeed, as Philip Abrams (1982: Ch. 1) describes, sociology began as a discipline in the nineteenth century in attempts to understand the historical processes involved in industrialization; thus history and sociology are engaged in the same enterprise. Both are concerned with two central questions: How does this thing we are concerned with come about? and, What are the best ways of describing what is taking place? The impact of the past on the present was an important theme for political and historical writing in the second half of the eighteenth century on the historical development of social institutions; and Marx took up this theme and expanded it in his analysis of capitalism; the rule of capital is 'the domination of living men by dead matter' (Bottomore and Rubel 1963: 19–21). Thus sociology should not just put investigations in their historical contexts, but should integrate historical forces as part of interactive agency-and-structure activity: 'society must be understood as a process constructed historically by individuals who are constructed historically by society' (Abrams 1982: 227).

Abrams (1982: xvii–xviii) quotes with approval from Anthony Giddens' then just published *Central Problems in Social Theory* (1979); he credits Giddens with reintroducing time as a central (but at that time neglected) concept in sociology, by emphasizing 'the sedimentation of institutional forms in long-term processes of social development' (Giddens 1979: 7). If we recover temporality as integral to social theory, then 'there simply are no logical or even methodological distinctions between the social sciences and history appropriately conceived' (1979: 230). This work of integrating history into social theory must include considering temporality in relation to the duality of agency and structure (1979: Ch. 6).

Giddens' structuration theory (1979, 1984) has provided an influential attempt to come to terms with agency and structure problems, by proposing that they are not separate and somewhat opposed entities, but intimately and deeply implicated in each other; structures are both the medium and the outcome of human activity; while much of social life is 'recursive' (reproductive rather than transformative) yet agents may be so-called in that they have the ability, the power, to make a difference in the social world. His scheme has great advantages, in detailing the implicated character of agency and structure, but it is also problematic. At common-sense level, and given longstanding traditions of thought, it is very hard to think of the social world without identifying heavy constraints and pressures from established institutions (Abrams 1982: 227), and especially hard if one is concerned (as in this book) with a minority social group. Giddens' theory does seem to overstate the power of people to make a difference, and to understate social constraint or limitation (Craib 1992: 120–2; Layder 1997: 164–70).

Critical realism

The respective characters of structures and agents have been analysed by the critical realists, who have also mounted critiques of Giddens (e.g. Archer

1982, 1998: 79); and have reacted against postmodernisms with their emphasis on present-day transactions – discourses, insubstantiality and uncertainties. Critical realists provide a convincing and usable analysis of ontological distinctions between agency and structure, which fully takes account of historical processes and of relationality.

Roy Bhaskar's argument is set out in *The Possibility of Naturalism* (1979: Ch. 2, esp. 42–7). This is a materialist argument, building on Marx's work in refining and discussing agency/structure issues. Bhaskar argues that sociology is concerned with persistent relations between individuals and groups and with relations between relations (1979: 36). Crucially, he argues, people and society 'do not constitute two moments of the same process. Rather they refer to radically different kinds of thing' (1979: 42) (so he disagrees with Giddens, who proposes they are part of the same 'moment', the duality of structure). Society has ontological depth; it would not exist without human activity, but people do not now in the present create it; they reproduce or transform it. For instance, we cannot speak without using existing means of communication, make without using existing materials or act except in some already existing context. This, he says, is an Aristotelian conception of human activity, where the paradigm is that of the sculptor who fashions a product out of the material and tools available: 'it is a transformational model of social activity' (Bhaskar 1979: 43).

The critical realist account builds in a historical dimension to both agency and society. Human activity (unlike societies) is characterized by intentionality; reasons, purposes, plans, comments on past activity, monitoring of activity. Societies have material continuity – that is, they have levels of existence drawn from past interrelations with agents. This account is essentially relational; the argument is that we have to be concerned most importantly with enduring relationships between social positions. Thus we should focus, for instance, not only on the child and adult, but on the social position of student in relation to that of teacher and in relation to the sedimented education system. Further we must consider relations between relations. An example might be: if child–adult relations are characterized by obedience and authority, we should then study relationships between these two concepts – how they intersect and are reproduced and transformed.

On the issue of process: how structures are reproduced and transformed, Bhaskar gives examples: in general people unconsciously reproduce structures; they marry and do paid work for their own purposes, but in so doing they reproduce marriage and the capitalist economy. When structures change – when people transform them – the explanation does not usually lie in people's intentions (though they may aim to change structures), it is an unintentional outcome of what they do (1979: 44). He summarizes his argument:

The model of the society/person I am proposing could be summarised as follows: people do not create society. For it always pre-exists them and is a necessary condition for their activity. Rather society must be regarded as an ensemble of structures, practices and conventions which individuals reproduce or transform, but which would not exist unless they did so. Society does not exist independently of human activity (the error of reification) but it is not the product of it (the error of voluntarism).

(Bhaskar 1979: 45–6)

Thus he proposes a model of the society/person connection, where there is an emphasis on material continuity, with reproduction and transformation providing for continuity and change – and hence of history (1979: 46–7). Bhaskar, drawing on the materialist tradition, pays tribute throughout his exposition to the comparable version of this conception of history set out by Marx and Engels:

History is nothing but the succession of the separate generations, each of which exploits the material, the capital funds, the productive forces handed down to it by all preceding generations, and thus, on the one hand, continues the traditional activity in completely changed circumstances and, on the other, modifies the old circumstances with a completely changed activity (Marx and Engels, 1970: 57).[1]

Layder further explains Bhaskar's arguments and their links with Marxism:

On the one hand, forms of agency represent the transformative capacities of individuals and groups as they come to terms with and alter the social circumstances they encounter in their everyday lives. On the other hand, systemic or structural aspects represent the historically formed standing conditions transmitted and inherited from the past (see Marx and Engels 1968: 96) which confront people as constraints and (enablements).

(Layder 1998b: 88)

These interactive processes are analysed by Margaret Archer (1998: 82–4). She proposes a three-stage agency/structure interaction cycle. At the first stage, we have *structural conditioning*, within which systemic properties can be understood as:

the emergent or aggregate consequences of past actions. Once they have been elaborated over time they are held to exert a causal influence upon subsequent interaction. Fundamentally they do so by shaping the situations in which later 'generations' of agents find themselves and by endowing various agents with different vested interests according to the positions they occupy in the structures they 'inherit' (in the class structure, in the social distribution of resources or in the educational system for example).

(Archer 1998: 82–3)

Stage two – *social interaction* – is structurally conditioned but never structurally determined, 'since agents possess their own irreducible emergent powers' (Archer 1998: 83). People may seek to pursue structural change or to maintain structural stability. As a result of the interaction, stage three – *structural elaboration* – takes place; though people may have aimed at certain goals (change or stability) the elaboration that takes place is the product of different outcomes pursued simultaneously by various social groups, and is largely unintended. This account of process gives due weight to the continued impact over time of both structure and agency on each other. The realist accepts that the results of past actions (structures) have effects as constraining or facilitating influences on agents which are not reducible or attributable to the practices of other contemporary agents.

Critical realism faces up to theoretical and empirical research problems. It gives a clear account of ontological distinctions between agency and structure, and shows how reproduction and transformation processes take place. It gives due place to the force of history in laying down sediments – as to both agents and structures. It takes account of power, vested interest, cultural capital; and shows both the limitations and possibilities of agency, including the agency of minorities. I think it provides useful guidelines to approaching the social study of childhood.

Generation

At this point, and within this broad relational approach to processes of the constituting of the social order, we can focus on generation as a key concept for studying childhood. I think there are two main enterprises. The first is to consider processes through which childhood is constructed and modified; that is to deploy and explore generationing processes through which childhood comes to have characteristics distinguishing it from adulthood. These generationing processes can take place at the four levels outlined earlier: in individual transactions between children and adults; in group transactions, as between pupils and teachers; in individual relations between people born at different points in history; in social policies handed down from an earlier cohort to a later one. The second enterprise is to consider the extent to which people can be said to inhabit a generation, to regard themselves as generationally positioned, even sharing certain ideas, and perhaps thinking of their generation as different from that of older social groups.[2]

As I noted earlier, to use the concept 'generationing' is, among other things, an extrapolation from women's use of 'gendering'. In the case of relations between women and men, womanhood and manhood, exploration of gender issues has served to uncover and also to problematize the processes whereby women and womanhood have been and are defined in contradistinction to men and manhood.[3] Study of these processes can be carried out at individual level and linked up to group levels; the way a woman experiences her relationships with men can be better understood if viewed as produced by larger-scale processes. In the case of children and childhood, we may start perhaps with what for most children is the first set of relationships – with their parents. The social positions of motherhood, fatherhood and childhood have their specific qualities in interrelation with each other, but they have been produced and are still being modified by larger-scale understandings of those positions and their interrelations. An example is given in Chapter 4, where parents reflect on the relevance of their own childhoods to their relations and interactions with their own children now. In Chapter 5, I explore relations between childhood and 'teacherhood' which take place at individual and group levels, but which change in the light of government policies on education. Another way of looking at processes in these generationed relations is through study of distinctions between received notions of childhood and experience.[4] In my most recent study (Childhood Study) I started by asking children to describe and discuss motherhood, fatherhood and childhood. Then I encouraged them to describe and discuss their daily lives and experiences. Both these methods allowed them to reflect on differences between received, categorical notions of those social positions (Connell 1987: 54–61) and how children and parents operationalize daily life, which may somewhat diverge from established notions of the social positions and relationships between them (for discussion of these points, see Alanen 2000).[5] Thus, through moving from taken-for-granted understandings, to study of processes whereby social positions and relations between them are constituted and transformed, the research enterprise moves towards relational sociology, as suggested by the critical realists.

The second main arena in which one may deploy the concept generation is through consideration of the extent of commonality that exists between people subject to the same or similar forces, influences, events. Mannheim (1952) – who is generally credited with the first comprehensive study of generation (for reviews see Pilcher 1994; Corsten 1999) – approached 'the problem of generation' in his study of the history of culture and in particular with a view to providing a theory of changes within and to culture. He analyses the formation of generations as taking place in three stages, called status or *location*, *actuality* and *unit* (Mannheim 1952: 302–7). People born (or located) in the same period of social and historical time within a society are exposed to a specific range of social, historical and political events and ideas, but their exposure – the opportunities and constraints for thought, experience and action – will vary according to their social class position. A group of young people become an actual generation 'in so far as they participate in the characteristic social and intellectual currents of their society and period' (1952: 304). Some members of an actual generation may establish a set of shared projects and goals; such a group forms a generational unit. An example might be the Impressionist painters in nineteenth-century France. As the generations move through the lifecycle they carry with them ideas rooted in those early exposures, and these ideas will be more or less defined and refined depending on which stage they as individuals and groups reached (location, actuality, unit). Writing in 1928, Mannheim may be forgiven for not taking account of gender, but his theory can encompass insights from feminist work; the character of people's exposure to cultural and political trends, and their ability to participate in social and intellectual currents, will differ according to gender.

Bourdieu provides an analysis (1986) of ways in which an elite generation reproduces itself. His focus is on the education system, and he develops the notion of *cultural capital* to discuss how adult elites transmit cultural knowledge, attitudes and behaviour to their children so that they will succeed in an education system structured by that same elite. In the education system of the UK, structured by social class divisions, this idea has clear relevance (see Chapter 5 for discussion). Bourdieu is pointing to the power of one generation to influence the next, as well as to retain control, especially within and through education. Though he does not emphasize process in the sense of interaction, he nevertheless points in more general terms to influence; the notion of habitus, with its connotations of dispositions acquired over time, has some resonances with the critical realist approach.

Study of the concept of generation is clearly centrally concerned with processes of continuity and change, how the past feeds into the present and on into the future, through the agency of people born and learning at certain periods of time. Michael Corsten (1999) usefully picks up the distinction introduced by Joan Robinson (1963) between logical time and historical time. Logical time is the outline of linear progress of time-points distinctly succeeding each other; historical time refers to a sequence of social events. Generational experience and understanding comprises intersecting components: the sequence of social events in historical time; the biographical development of individuals, and the coalescence into groups of people who share some orientations and knowledge, but may differ for instance as to birth date, specific experience and response to events. For Corsten, a generation of people have a sense of belonging – they not only share assumptions, they also share a sense that other people share similar assumptions. This argument gets rid of the idea of cohorts based on age and focuses instead on shared assumptions among people of somewhat varying birth dates.

This point is also made by Abrams (1982: Ch. 8) who argues that identity is made within the 'double construction of time' – where life history and world history coalesce to transform each other. Where there is an unchanged social world, unchanged system of meanings and possibilities (as in a 'traditional' society), then a sociological generation may encompass many biological generations. Abrams bases his argument partly on Erikson's vision (1968) of psychological development through fixed stages, so that identity is structured psychologically as well as through social interaction. One might want to comment that a more thorough-going sociological proposition would be that even where there is no dramatic change in social events/currents/beliefs, identities will change over time because of the build-up of intersections between people and social structures. Bourdieu makes a useful contribution with the idea of the *social generation*, not firmly linked to age cohort. Though, on the one hand, (in *Sociology in Question*, 1993) he seems to focus on cohorts of real people passing through time, on the other hand and more interestingly, he proposes elsewhere generation as a category for structuring social relations. Thus in *Homo Academicus* (1988), he sees generations as socially constructed through power relations. This kind of approach allows for the idea that people may identify with a generation which is not theirs in terms of the time when they were born or grew up. For instance, some people may identify with the '1960s generation' even though they were born much later in chronological time. In thinking about UK society, this is a useful idea. Thus people born in another country but making their way in the UK may carry with them and deploy some elements of the country-of-origin culture, but may also forge a new generational culture in the UK, which is linked both to their time-of-birth-cohort and to the social experiences of migration and contact with UK social institutions and cultures. Ethnic minority parents' and children's negotiations of homework (Chapter 5: 82), and Muslim girls' visions of their futures (Chapter 7: 130) provide examples where these issues are in play.

Conceptualizing childhood

In this chapter I have focused on ideas that seem to me useful in considering the social condition of childhood and childhood as an intergenerational relational category. Here I review the main ways in which these ideas help us to conceptualize and study childhood.

History

Incorporating history into analysis of the social order seems essential to understanding how it comes about that we have certain specific childhoods. It is an immediately acceptable idea that the past influences the present, that we cannot operate except through established tools. In particular if we are considering any social group which is subordinated within the social order, then it seems crucial to take account of the weight of the past bearing down on the group's social position and its ability to negotiate, improve or transform.

If we take it that children constitute a minority social group, then consideration of the legacies of history seems particularly appropriate. This is the main topic in Chapter 8, which considers how to account for differences between Finnish and UK childhoods, and points to the continued relevance of the social history of the two countries. Throughout Chapters 4 to 7, it emerges that rights are a central concern for children. By taking seriously both the impacts of history on the structural positioning of children and childhood, and children's understandings, we may try to contribute to raising the status of childhood. Of especial interest, as regards children growing up in the UK today, are longstanding gendered understandings of childhood and adulthood. These chapters will explore the extent to which present-day children's experiences and their agency relates to these understandings and how far such ideas are becoming modified or transformed.

Agency and structure – critical realism

The separation of agency and structure into ontologically distinct entities, as set out in critical realism, provides a firm basis for consideration of childhood as relational category. This separation focuses attention on the distinctive features of *structures*: the ideologies, policies, established practices regarding childhood and the power these have – mediated through adult power – over childhood. In this book I have considered two major sites or institutions where, children tell me, they live their daily lives – the home (Chapter 4) and school (Chapter 5), and tried to show how longstanding and more recent ideologies, policies and social practices control children's lives, and how the agency of both children and adults is implicated, through their interrelations, to reproduce or modify childhoods.

On *agency*, critical realism identifies motivating forces stretching from the past into the future: established dispositions, reasons and experiences, feelings on the day, wishes and goals for the future. This analysis is useful again in drawing attention to processes across time, and in providing a method for considering children's experiences and encounters with adults and other children. (Later examples are Stuart's story, Chapter 5: 83 and

Sandra's story, Chapter 6: 90) Of interest, too, is how children constitute themselves as a social group – through discussing and defining their common experiences over time in relation to adult social groups, their present experience of child–adult relations, and their wishes for modification of these (Chapters 6 and 7).

Generation

In various respects childhood can be well understood through generational perspectives. First, we can use the idea of generationing (analogously to gendering) as a concept that helps us understand processes through which social positions are constituted, reproduced and transformed through relational activity. Study of generationing is essential because childhood is essentially relational with adulthood, not least because the power to define it lies with adults, who define it as different from adulthood. Children are in no doubt that childhood differs from adulthood.

Second, I have suggested that Mannheim's concept of generation, and as reconsidered by others, is useful on several counts. In his formulation, it allows us to understand groups of people as constituting three levels of generational affiliation: as people located historically and socially at a particular time, as an actual generation who participate in social events; and as a unit who think and work together. The concept of generation brings into play processes of continuity and change in the social world. It further enables us to conceptualize 'the double construction of time' – the intertwining of individual or group history with world history. Thus the concept of generation brings to the study of childhood a historical perspective at small-scale and large-scale levels.

Bourdieu usefully proposes the 'social generation', where groups of people share similar experiences (for instance of migration, war, education policies) which influence their later experiences and relationships. The notion of social generation thus defined helps to deal with one of the problems with studying childhood; that is, how to cope with the large differences we (have been taught to) observe between very small children and 'children' aged, say, 17. (Under-18s are children in the UNCRC).[6] The notion of generation allows both children and adults to associate these developmentally disparate people under the umbrella of or 'this generation of children', living within a specific set of social conditions, and subject to specific understandings of childhood.

Bourdieu's points (1986) on cultural capital are also relevant, for instance for understanding the UK's current divided and divisive education system; as Chapter 5 (p. 69) argues, social and political elites have maintained the power to transmit cultural capital through private schools. The notion of the transmission of cultural capital also helps us understand how and why some social groups of children conform more than others to the education system. For instance, Muslim parents teach their children obedience, deference and hard work; this fits well with how teachers expect children to behave nowadays, and Muslim children seem to do well at school. Other groups of children, whose parents do not inculcate such attitudes and behaviour, may find the education system less acceptable, and may do worse.

Thus focusing on historical issues in sociological thought helps us understand childhood. The social relations of agency and structure require children to work with and against structures with 'ontological depth', with characteristics rooted in the past, such as ideas about childhood, education, parent–child relationships. As a generation, children take on board notions of shared social status and shared experience with people at differing stages of childhood, but all living through childhoods as understood at a specific period of historical time in a given society.

Finally, the discussion in this and the previous chapter points to the importance of keeping both gender and generation in play. Study of childhood, on the arguments I have considered, requires analysis of the relations of ruling, including the division of labour. We have to look at intergenerational gendered relations, for instance, the ways in which women and girls, and women and boys are socially positioned and interrelate within households and schools where the power lies elsewhere. The concept of the intermediate domain is useful here for exploring children's and women's people work. One feature of this study must be changes in these relationships, and in child and adult expectations according to social stage and ethnicity. Thus both children and adults have changing expectations and understanding of childhood once children take the social steps from primary to secondary school. Girls in some ethnic groups find themselves understood differently by parents once they reach puberty, as regards their contributions to household and school labour. Keeping a clear line of argument, faced with gender, generation, social stage and ethnicity, is one of the difficult tasks of this book.

4 | Relations with parents

This chapter considers young people's accounts of childhood in its relations with parenthood.[1] The main aim is not to present data on how they understand their social position, but more precisely to consider how such understandings get established and how they – and adults' understandings – intersect to constitute, reproduce and transform childhoods. So I shall not set out 'findings' for their own sake, but rather use young people's accounts, in various ways, to analyse relational processes.

Child–parent relations in social context

The first focus is on processes through which the physical and social conditions of childhoods and parents' interpretations of these shape children's daily lives. Rather than give snippets from many accounts, I give here an extensive quotation from one 9-year-old's account (Childhood Study, North Primary). Gamse lives with her parents and four sibs in a two-bedroomed council flat. Both parents are busy: with childcare and running a shop. Out of school time, she spends her time with her immediate family or with other relatives; she is not allowed to play out, because her parents think the local children rough.

Interviewer: So what do you do outside school, after school?

Gamse: Sometimes I just stay at home and just look after the twins [aged 1 year] and help my Mum, or I might go out to my cousins' or my uncle's, or I might go to the shop which is my Dad's shop, sometimes I go there.

Interviewer: With someone?

Gamse: I either go with my Mum and my sister [aged 6] and the twins, or I go with my Dad.

Interviewer: So most of your time you spend with your family?

Gamse: Mostly I spend it with my family [meaning nuclear family]. Before, I used to go to my cousins a lot and my uncle a lot. But now that my Dad's got a new business I mostly stay with them, because my Mum's got a lot of things to do at home, and my Dad's got a lot to do at the shop. Or sometimes my Mum goes into the shop.

Interviewer: So is he working longer hours?

Gamse: Well, he used to work, he works from seven to nine at night. But they take turns to be in the shop, or sometimes my, both of them have to be in the shop and then we go down there. They have to take us with them. Downstairs there's a little room where we stay and play games, or we just watch TV or a video . . .

Interviewer: Space and time [I am referring to the topic list] – do you have enough time to do things and space to do them? Basically, do you have a good day?

Gamse: Yes, mostly I have a good day. Sometimes my brother [aged 12] gets on my nerves and teases me and starts punching me and that. It's really horrible.

Interviewer: How often is that?

Gamse: Not often, only when he's had a really bad day. Most of the time he's in a really good mood and he doesn't tease me.

Interviewer: And do you share a room with –

Gamse: Yes, I do. Because I live in a small flat. My brother has his own room, it's very small and you can't even fit in. My Mum and Dad sleep on the sofa bed in the sitting room, and me and my sister sleep in bunk beds and the twins in their cots in my bedroom as well.

Interviewer: Does that work out OK?

Gamse: Yes, it works out fine. I would prefer the sofa bed. Sometimes when my Dad comes home late, I get in there, and then when he comes I get in my own bed.

Interviewer: Health [referring to the topic list] – is it your job to stay healthy?

Gamse: Yes, it is actually, cos sometimes I go out with my brother shopping, and get some vegetables or something. And I don't go to Woolworth's to get some sweets! And, or sometimes –

Interviewer: It's up to you to decide whether to buy sweets?

Gamse: No, it's up to my Mum, but mostly it's my Mum – and Dad. They want me to keep healthy and everything. I can't explain it.

Interviewer: Do you think it's more they look after you?

Gamse: Well, I look after myself half the time, but mostly it's my Mum looks after me – makes sure I eat the right things. Like veg or sometimes meat and not much fizzy drinks. Water, at dinnertime – we have to drink two glasses of water and then have a fizzy drink. So we're not allowed to have a fizzy drink first.

Interviewer: Are there other sorts of rules round your house?

Gamse: One is not to tease, and to be helpful to each other, but that's only when my brother gets in a bad mood. Or there's to help each other, like when my Mum says do something, you have to do it, not say, No, I don't want to do it. And really that's –

Interviewer: And apart from looking after the twins, is there anything else you do?

Gamse: Yes, in the morning, I'm responsible for waking my sister up. My brother wakes himself up, cos 8 o'clock he goes to school, and in the morning my Mum sleeps. So it's my responsibility to wake up and wake Mary up and get her breakfast and get herself ready. But mostly she does it herself, cos I make the breakfast and wake her up and –

Interviewer: Cos your Mum would be looking after the twins and your Dad down at the shop?

Gamse: Yes.

Gamse's daily life is structured through the family's housing and the busy working lives of both parents, mediated by her parents' decisions on how childhood should be lived in the local context. They think the outside world is not an appropriate place for her, and that adult supervision is essential at all times. It seems the parents have made clear to the children their values and norms for family life; and the parents are in authority over the behaviour of their children.

More generally, her account points to broad sociophysical factors, operating across time, which structure all the young people's lives. The character and quality of their daily lives are strongly related to type and quality of housing and to parental work-hours; thus parents' fortunes influence the next generation. Wider social forces influence parents' control over their children's days; the hostile character of outside space influences parental responses in the shape of supervision and restriction. Relational processes work downwards from large-scale trends, mediated by parental behaviour, to shape children's lives.

Characterizing child–parent relations

The relational character of young people's understandings can be explored in a number of ways. Here I set out first a summary of the main points made by my informants, aged 5–13 years, from three studies.[2] These points emerge both from direct questioning about the statuses of child and parent, and from elicited accounts of and reflections on daily life. There is considerable commonality in how they talk about and experience childhood, hinged on their understanding that childhood is relational with parenthood. It is commonality across age, gender and ethnicity, although within that there are some differences.

Children and the family

One of the main characteristics of childhood offered by young people is its difference from parenthood. It is through living with parents that young people first learn that they inhabit the status of child. Parental definitions constitute them as children. Whilst, according to young people, these definitions vary somewhat between families, it is through their parents' behaviour that people learn to do childhoods.

According to the young people, child–parent relationships were gendered; mothers were in charge of day-to-day management of the home and children. Girls and boys of all ages report many more conversations with mothers than with fathers: discussions, getting permission, chatting, confiding, hearing about family history and relationships. Though some reported that their father was the ultimate moral authority, most provided evidence that mothers managed the household and interacted with children.

Most young people talked warmly about being and doing with 'the family'. They described family and the home as sources of material goods and of comfort, and of valued relationships. They enjoyed 'family times' and especially if their father took part (since a rarer occurrence?). These times included going out together, evenings at home together, wider family get-togethers and celebrations. A small minority of young people clearly lacked this comforting happy home life; they talked about adult cruelty, neglect, oppression and painful experiences of parental separation.

Gender and generation

Asked what kinds of things mothers and fathers do, young people gave normative accounts, drawing categorical distinctions between mothers and fathers. Mothers were responsible for the home and childcare, fathers for bringing in financial resources. In practice, these norms were broken when the mother was the sole parent, or where parents were splitting up, or where the father was unemployed.

In their accounts of daily life, young people expressed very little negative emotion towards mothers. As Edwards and Alldred (2000) also note, children accept mothers' anger and irritation, because they understand their mother's stressful lives and recognize that anger is contextualized within a basically loving relationship. Some of the younger children were in the process of coming to terms with family change – fathers moving out, stepfathers moving in, mothers coming to terms with lone parenthood – and they talked mainly in terms of process and practicalities. It was the older ones who expressed anger more against fathers – for failing to care about and support the family.[3]

Thus, for these samples, the mother was the most constant figure for the young people. Whether or not fathers were resident, she was 'there' for them, both in person and relationally, more than fathers, many of whom had very long hours of work. The domestic division of labour, structured by the relations of ruling, ensured her presence as homemaker, decisionmaker and carer, and as the person with whom the young people negotiated domestic activity at home, homework, free time, and time outside the home. It also shone through the data that young people appreciated having a confidant and for most of them this was their mother (cf. Ghate and Daniels 1997: Ch. 3).

The social status of women as principal carers ensured also that grandmothers were significant figures in their grandchildren's lives. Many of the families lived nearby to grandparents; some had over three generations 'always' lived in the area; some newer arrivals to the UK and London had grouped their three-generational – and extended – families in the same area. Interdependent relations included grandmothers' childcare work and grandparents' financial contributions to the family, and reciprocally children and parents phoning and calling round at grandparents' homes – keeping in touch, doing the shopping, providing meals.

Obedience, privilege and negotiation

Young people's accounts indicated that at home moral issues were faced, debated and resolved (see also Chapter 6). Parents rightly had authority over their children. Many young people also provided justification for parental authority – parents knew more than children and had a duty to protect them and provide for them; so it was for them to decide how life should be lived, including how children should behave. The accounts give many examples of parents setting out general precepts, as well as making practical decisions.

Unlike parents, children were free from major responsibilities. Childhood was a never-to-be-repeated time when you could enjoy this freedom. Indeed children had a right to 'free time', partly as a component of this absence of responsibility, and partly because much of the time they had to obey parental diktats.

Within the broad parameters of parental authority, young people reported that they aimed to exercise some control over activity. Families varied in how much scope there was for negotiation. Negotiation included: discussion, refusal to comply, bargaining, delaying tactics. The goals included: escape from unwelcome tasks, free time, time to continue with the activity in hand, escape from parental control, own control over use of time and space.

Apprenticeship and participation

Young people described childhood as including both learning and participation. In both, time present and time future were implicated. It was, importantly, a time of apprenticeship, which has three components. Children must learn how to be a good enough member of their family and must learn the cultural, and in some cases religious, customs and duties in which their family participates. They must work on the project of their own life – how best to juggle possibilities and constraints in the here and now. And they must learn at home and school what they need for adult life. Thus young people subscribed to the socialization thesis – childhood is in part preparation for adult life, and childhood is a journey during which one learns – but they also ascribed themselves agency in their own socialization.

Through their accounts of daily life, young people demonstrated their participation in the construction, maintenance and advancement of the family enterprise. By the age of 5 years, they were making important contributions to self-care (washing, dressing, monitoring thirst and hunger) and thus relieving their mothers of these tasks; and by 9 years they were mostly in charge of their own care. They contributed to the making and remaking of family relationships; this included maintaining contact with family members who lived elsewhere (such as fathers and grandparents). They took part in household maintenance through cleaning, clearing up, cooking. Through these three measures they contributed to the division of labour at home (for similar findings, see Brannen *et al.* 2000).

Dependence and interdependence

Children are highly dependent on their parents' material resources. In the UK, where there are gross inequalities in these resources, children's dependency is very obvious; the quality of their childhoods varies widely.[4] Even within my small-scale school-based studies, where the families all lived in a small radius, there were huge differences as to the quality of housing, the quality of the immediate neighbourhood, access to out-of-school learning and leisure facilities, the character of children's lives at home. In the neighbourhood-based Risk Study, wealthier parents and those with more cultural and social capital were better able to access and choose services and notably to choose secondary schools for their children; poorer parents and those new to the country were aware how disadvantaged they and their children were.

The young people were dependent on parents for money, for access to friends and to spaces and times outside the home. Many got pocket money, but in some cases only if they behaved well during the week, and parents restricted some children's spending choices. All of them, except some of the older boys, had to ask permission to go out, and most had to specify with whom and where, and when they would be back. Some girls were not allowed out at all, and many young people were restricted to a narrow area outside the home, or to friends' homes. Where they wished to go to leisure and sports centres or to special interest classes, parents commonly accompanied them by car or on foot. Some reported that they could not use such facilities because they were too expensive, or because parents' busy time-schedules could not stretch to chaperoning them.

These dependencies coexist with interdependencies. Most accounts show that young people both received from and gave love to their parents. Parental protection and provision was balanced by children's contributions to the domestic division of labour. In some families parents put high hopes on children's later contributions to the family, especially where parents had immigrated to the UK, were suffering hardship and looked to this next generation to better the family finances and support them later on. Young people in these families expressed their sense of gratitude to their parents – for their hard work and care – and explicitly recognized their own life-long responsibilities to their parents. These ideas were less prevalent among those young people (a minority) living in well-to-do native English families. But in all, their predominant emphasis was on interdependency rather than on independence, either as a goal for the future or now.

Some comments on these points

The foregoing paragraphs provide a broad account of group interrelationships, between children and parents. Some general points emerge. The first is that children's positioning – along dimensions of obedience and negotiation, apprenticeship and participation, dependence and interdependence – amounts to a conceptualization of the relational character of childhood.

And processes within that status relationship take place not just at the level of daily interaction but also at the level of social policies which define – whether purposefully or not – how childhood is to be dealt with. For the UK, childhood is understood mainly within family policies, and thus the characteristics of childhoods, as I noted, are heavily dependent on parental resources (see Chapter 8 for a contrasting set of understandings and policies).

Second, these accounts forcibly demonstrate young people's agency: in self-care, in the construction of family relationships, and in housework and childcare. In all these respects they are participating in people work: the interdependent enterprises whereby people accomplish the tasks needed to keep the family afloat. Children's work contributes both directly to the family enterprise and indirectly by freeing up adult time.

Third, these accounts draw attention to intersections of gender and generation. Traditional divisions of labour ensure that mothers are the mainstay of the home, there both physically and morally as the key parent, to whom her children relate. Grandmothers, more than grandfathers, figure as significant relatives. Relations were reciprocal across three generations.

Fourth, gender intersects with age or school status. Girls of all ages tended to be more restricted in use of public space than boys, but social status as a secondary school student freed up most young people somewhat, especially boys.

Fifth, running through the strands of young people's accounts is a rights agenda, especially focusing on the three Ps: protection, provision and participation. Though they did not talk explicitly about rights, except the right to free time, they emphasized parental duty to protect them and provide for them. As one said, being a child 'means you've got someone looking after you, and you know they're looking after you'. In practice, they thought parents provided what they could for their children. They varied in how far they felt they participated in decision-making on topics that affected them, along a continuum from those who thought parents made all the decisions, to those who claimed to make many themselves within a broad parent-organized framework. In general, they also accepted it as right that parents should have the final say.

Young people talk about child–parent relations – intersections of generation and gender

In this section, I give some examples of individual child–adult relations, drawn from 9-year-olds' accounts (in the Childhood Study), in order to explore variations in the specific ways that generationing and gendering processes construct childhoods.

First is Alan, whose parents came from war-torn far east country.

Interviewer: What kinds of things do your parents expect of you?

Alan: To be helpful and have a good life and have a happy time with my family. And my Mum wants me to help her a lot, and to be good at school and make friends so I have a happy life. And she's proud of me right now because I know how to do the violin and karate, so she's quite proud of me really.

(East Primary School, Year 5)

Later, in another session, he explained why his mother was urging him and his younger sister to do well:

Well, she wants me to get talented when I grow up, and she said that when she was young she didn't have the time to play anything, because there was a war going on and she had to look after her brothers and sisters because her mum and dad [were working] . . . And then she's not quite clever because she didn't go to school a lot once her mum got her to do the cooking and take the children to school.

He expressed sorrow and sympathy for his mother's childhood, and felt that he and his sister carried his mother's hopes for the future of the family. Later he said he tried to help his mother learn English and sometimes read books with her.

Alan's account indicates his close relations with his mother – his father (who was out for long hours at work) figures very little in his discourse. Gendered processes had ensured that his mother, as a girl, had been assigned childcare and household responsibilities. These processes work across the generations; she wanted his childhood to be better than hers, and his knowledge of it affected his understanding of his own childhood. He had also accepted his mother's wishes for his future, and had taken responsibility for reciprocating his mother's care by helping her make her way in this new country.

Another boy gave clear expression to a way of life where religious practice is integral to daily life.

Sajid: They expect me to be nice, good, clear up, and we have to pray to God every day five times, but we miss one [at school] so we pray four times. My Dad says I have to study a lot, and my Mum says you have to pray when you come back from school and learn. She tells me to learn a whole page by heart and that's really hard to do . . .

Interviewer: What else are children meant to do?

Sajid:	Be good. If you are a believer, you have to pray to God. I pray four times and the Holy Koran and that makes five times. Every weekend my Mum and Dad expect me to pray for three hours. So I can learn two pages by heart. That takes up quite a long time. Then when I'm ready, my Mum listens to me. But my Mum says, you have to do it proper and perfect, you should not get even one mistake. If you do make one mistake, you have to learn it all over again.
Interviewer:	Are there good things about being a child?
Sajid:	The good thing for me is, when I have free time I can play football.

(East Primary School, Year 5)

In this case, both parents acted to ensure the continuity across the generations of Islamic ways of life, but it was the mother who ensured that the relevant daily and weekly routines took place. And these intergenerational processes also intersected with the demands of a society where secular school takes up children's time. This boy had to fit school, mosque, language tuition classes, and the homework from each, into his day. He was among several Muslim boys who strikingly described childhood as hard, and put very high value on their small amounts of free time.

These two Muslim girls spoke with enthusiasm about learning and doing the household jobs appropriate for girls.

Interviewer:	What do parents expect of their children?
Rumena:	To be good and behave.
Sidra:	Yes, and they try to teach them discipline, so when they get older they can do the jobs parents do not, and learn them to do jobs. Like looking after things and clearing up.
Interviewer:	Anything else?
Rumena:	How to live.
Interviewer:	Meaning?
Rumena:	Not letting mice and rats into your home and clearing up your bedroom. We find it boring doing all that stuff and when we're mums having to do all that clearing up of our rooms, it'll be even harder.
Sidra:	I want to be a mother, but I also want to work, to be an optician. I like doing stuff about eyes and my Dad says I can.
Interviewer:	Do you think of yourselves as children?
Sidra:	Yes. You don't have so much responsibility. You don't have to do much like getting food ready. They [parents] do all the hard things.

Rumena: I do baking – cakes and biscuits – not cooking. Your parents pay for you – at theme parks.

Interviewer: And what do you do?

Rumena: We get pocket money.

Interviewer: What do you use it for?

Rumena: We use the money for the right things.

Interviewer: What are they?

Sidra: Sweets and things.

Interviewer: And are you living the life you want to lead?

Rumena: Yes.

Sidra: Yes [great enthusiasm from both girls].

Interviewer: And has life changed at all recently?

Rumena: Yes, since I've turned 10, I've got more responsibility. I've got to learn to do things that my Mum does. You have to learn more things.

Sidra: My Mum does the cooking. But I clean the house, put the washing in the machine and learn a lot of stuff for the future . . .

[Section about brother who has a very hard life – with school work and mosque work, and the parents are very 'hard' on him.]

Interviewer: So do you think your mother and father are strict?

Sidra: No. No, only to my brother. But if you do something wrong, there's no offence in them giving you a whack. Then I start laughing and she starts laughing and she runs after me and you just, it's like a joke.

(East Primary School, Year 5)

These two girls had a clear, gendered, understanding of how their life now and in the future should be lived, based on Islamic teaching. They both went to the mosque each day after school, like the boys, but religious observance for girls took up less time, since they did not have to learn the Koran, but only to read it and learn about Islam.

The intersections of gender and generation in their lives allowed these girls to experience their current lives, including their domestic responsibilities, as both acceptable and pleasurable. They were already aware that later on issues of career versus traditional women's roles might have to be dealt with, but at present they did not identify conflicts. For the 12-year-olds, these issues were becoming more important (for discussion see Chapter 5: 82).

These four young people, whose parents had immigrated from widely differing societies, shared a common understanding: that their parents had a clear vision of their children's future lives. This vision comprised generational processes mediated by gender. The kin relations of children to parents were to continue when children became adults, with gendered responsibilities to the family negotiated in relation to the sociopolitical context of UK society. All the boys and girls whose parents had immigrated – from middle eastern countries, the far east and the Indian subcontinent – expressed very strong commitment to their families. This included learning their mother tongue in order to communicate with older family members who knew little English, and to ensure cultural continuity from those earlier generations through their own. Similarly they shared with their parents deep concern for the well-being of family in the country of origin, with letters and phone calls and hopes and plans for visits featuring in their accounts.

In contrast to the above accounts, some of the young people were living lives which approximated to traditional English models of childhood, structured within also traditional gendered parental lives. For instance, Simon's father was out most of the day in a professional job, and his mother had a part-time job locally which allowed her to accompany her son and daughter to and from school. He had a protected childhood, in which he thought his time out of school was essentially free for him to do as he pleased, though mainly at home, where his mother was based.

> *Simon:* After school – sometimes I invite a friend round, or I go to a friend's, or I just go home and read [he details the names and authors of novels he is reading] ... And on Tuesdays I do art class and that's all I do ...
>
> *Interviewer:* So in your day do you have enough time and space to do what you want to do?
>
> *Simon:* Yes.
>
> *Interviewer:* Some children get lots of homework these days.
>
> *Simon:* We don't get much homework, only at weekends ...
>
> *Interviewer:* Do your parents expect things from you, to do or to be?
>
> *Simon:* Not really, no. Well, yes, I suppose so.
>
> *Interviewer:* Some people say they have jobs.
>
> *Simon:* Well, um, yes, I think I do actually. Because on, on Wednesday, I have to tidy my room and um, on Monday I have to get everything ready for the week, PE kit and –
>
> *Interviewer:* And apart from now, do you think they have ideas about what they want for you in the longer term?
>
> *Simon:* They want me to do well at school, and go to a good secondary school.
>
> (North Primary School, Year 5)

Simon's account contrasts with those quoted earlier. He did not readily express understanding of his parents' models of childhood, and I had to prompt him (on homework, housework and the future) to fill in the picture of his days. He thought his activities out of school were for him to determine, within the clear understanding that he could not go out alone, but no doubt his childhood was structured through unspoken parental ideas that childhood should be free and protected and unpressurized. Having a well-resourced home made this possible. Like most of the children, his account shows that his main day-to-day relationship across the generations was with his mother. Unlike many children of immigrants, who knew their parents had clear ideas about their future jobs and lives, this boy's understanding stretched merely as far as knowing that his parents would like him to go to a 'good' secondary school.

Jan belonged to a family of women; her father lived elsewhere, but sometimes 'stayed over'; she lived sometimes with her mother and brother (1 year old), and sometimes at her grandmother's nearby; she stayed there some nights so that her mother was free to go out with friends. Her mother had a semi-professional job, but was now at home with the young boy. Jan explained that she did not go to classes out of school, partly because the family could not afford them.

> *Interviewer*: And do you have any jobs?
>
> *Jan*: Yes, um look after my brother, and sometimes I cook. I've only learned to cook potatoes and spaghetti bolognese and . . . clean the stairs and that's all the jobs I've got.
>
> *Interviewer*: So do you reckon you have enough time to do things you want?
>
> *Jan*: I do do things I want to. Cos on Wednesday and Friday I go to a club. [She describes the club and also explains she does gym and dance at school.]
>
> *Interviewer*: And would you say you expect anything from your Mum, or your Nan or your Dad?
>
> *Jan*: My Mum does enough for me, because she takes me out, and so does my Dad. And my Nan – she takes me out and does a lot of things with me. And all I want from them is love and respect.
>
> *Interviewer*: Yes, and do you get that?
>
> *Jan*: Yes.
>
> (North Primary School, Year 5)

Jan's account indicates that in her family women and girls openly discussed together gender issues. She knew her grandmother's and mother's history and that of other women in the family. On another occasion, she and a friend told me about the disadvantages their mothers had discussed with them of pregnancy as a teenager. Like Simon, she did not think her parents had clear plans and purposes for her future life. Indeed her mother 'wants me to be what I want to be'. She herself, through conversations with one of her aunts, who was training to be a lawyer, had become interested in legal training too. So across the generations, in this family, girls learned to weigh up possibilities and choices in the light of family history.

Parents talk about childhood

Next I consider generational processes implicated in how parents discuss child–parent relations, and notably how they understand their own parental tasks and responsibilities. Parents (in the Greenstreet and Risk Studies) regarded themselves as responsible for the character and quality of their children's childhoods. They aimed to 'give' their children adequate childhoods. In this they allied themselves theoretically with the notion that parents structure childhoods; and that, within those broad structures, children and parents negotiate the precise and changing character of daily life and experience. Underlying these notions of parental responsibility is an understanding that the state does not carry a major responsibility for the welfare of children, and indeed many parents in my studies were extremely critical of poor services for children, and especially of the education service.[5]

In thinking about their children's lives, parents commonly call on their memories of their own childhoods (cf. Scott 2000; Thomson et al. 2000). People are said to 'narrativize' their experiences of the world and their own role in it (Bruner 1990: Ch. 4). In common, across social class, ethnicity and country of birth, parents in our studies recalled freedom to explore, a safe clean environment, and the absence of the need for constant parental supervision. This mother, who moved as an adult to London from a north European country, speaks for many parents.[6]

> *Interviewer*: What's life like for parents and children round here?
> *Mother*: I think it's very difficult, it's very dangerous. Before, in my country, it was more safe. It's – children can walk to school by themselves, they can play by themselves, but here it's not possible really. You have to watch them all the time. The crime around – I think the situation isn't very good . . . Pollution also, a lot of cars round everywhere. When I was her age, I think I remember my childhood was very nice. I was free, I think. I mean many things I could do without my parents watching me. They did watch us but it wasn't like – I didn't feel scared. But I think we talk to children about, you know, all this kidnapping and things like that, and they are – they don't feel free.

Two principal fears for childhoods now ran through parental accounts: stranger danger and traffic danger. These together necessitated constant supervision and fear, and also required teaching children to be careful and fearful. Within these broad parameters, parents gave specific, somewhat varying accounts. A key topic was a comparison between their own and their children's childhoods. Past childhoods were freer, but those who had had rural childhoods described them as exceptionally free even compared to city life at the time. Parents' childhoods, and especially in some other societies, were characterized by respect for elders, and parental discipline was important in socializing children. Some mothers described childhoods lived in poverty and under harsh parental discipline; they aimed to ensure that the bad old days were not repeated for their own children. Parents also described community responsibility – 'looking out for children' – as a feature of past childhoods in the UK and other societies. I quote here from a father reflecting on the relationship between his own childhood experiences and his 4-year-old daughter's childhood now.[7]

Father: For me it's slightly different from even her, because she was born in this country whereas myself as a kid I was born in the West Indies, and that's in the 50s, early 50s. So when I was growing up, it's a lot different from now because, even the way in which they, the role, the system play in the authority parents have in bringing up their children and disciplining their children. In the West Indies when I was a young boy, I couldn't really, like if I was walking down the road and I saw an elder, whether it would be someone I know or somebody I've seen for the first time in my life, I feel I had to show respect to them by saying, Good afternoon, Sir, or Good afternoon, Ma'am. Kids nowadays pass. It's a different way, here in this country it's totally different from what we knew in the West Indies in those times. People pass one another and it's like they don't acknowledge one another; it's not like that – it wasn't like that in those times. You know, in my time as a youth growing up, different. And parents discipline children as they sees fit. You know, like if they feel it's necessary to discipline a child because of his behaviour they do it, and the system would not really, unless someone really took extreme measures and abused their children. But over here is different. For instance, if one of these kids did something terrible, and I decided to give him a few straps, and then he ended up with marks on him, he went to school and the social worker sees the marks on him, then I'll be in trouble. You see what I'm saying. In the West Indies you'd get a good hiding, you get marks, then the teacher knows you got the marks because you did something you shouldn't do and you know you got disciplined for it. Even the teachers in the school they used to discipline children, with strap in school. A different thing.

Interviewer: It sounds a bit like you're saying there was more respect, between parents and children?

Father: Oh yes, the kids, people grew up with more respect in my time, you know, than kids nowadays. Because the things children would come out with, well, these ones [that is, his own children] are not allowed to be like that because I still try to make sure they get as much of the discipline as I got in my time. When they're round me they have to have certain discipline.

Later he explained why children have to be restricted to playing indoors:

Where I come from, from the time you're 3 years, 4 years old, you're outside playing, and people just – it's everybody's responsibility . . . to make sure these kids are safe . . . and don't have accidents and things like that, people always looking out for that. But sometimes in this country you might have neighbours and they see the kids playing and see the kids getting out of hand and they don't, they don't really busy themselves, because as far as they're concerned it's not their kids.

He then gave an example where a neighbour cursed the 4-year-old for bad behaviour on the street (in London). The neighbour should have come and discussed the child's behaviour with him and he could then have disciplined the child. He thought that having to restrict children to the home led to rebelliousness, and problems between children and parents.

This father was facing a society where, from his point of view, the necessary basis of the social contract between adults and children had broken down. Children's respect for adults, adult duty to discipline children, and community responsibility for children's behaviour had given way to individual parent–child relations where there were no adequate sanctions to socialize children; furthermore, traffic and strangers meant children's active play was curtailed. He could not behave as he thought a father should, and his children's lives were damaged by the social and physical environment. Thus his construction of childhoods now, in London, was negative by comparison with his own, and he did not identify ways of improving these childhoods. Later the interviewer asked if he thought childhoods today were in any way better than when he was a child. He answered, 'No, for then you could always get a job' – and now getting a good job depended so much on access to good education; mass media exposed children to violence, and a culture of drugs and crime surrounded them.

Given the restrictions they thought they should impose on their children's freedom to roam in the public world, many parents thought they should compensate, by providing children with supervised access to a social life with friends, and to outside space – in parks and on trips; also that they should provide opportunities for physical exercise through organized sports and other activities. Parents also accompanied their children on journeys to their friends out of school time.

An example of how parents and children come to terms with the significance of past childhoods when considering how young people should do childhood now is given by a Greenstreet mother and daughter aged 10.[8] Before this excerpt, they have been talking with me about how far Jane takes responsibility for looking after herself and contributing to household maintenance.

Interviewer: So are you happy with the division of responsibility between her and you? Do you wish she would do more, or less, or are you happy?

Mother: Certainly it's very different from when I was a child. I mean – when I was 5 I used to go to school on a bus to a school that was three miles away.

Interviewer: In this country?

Mother: Yes. In some ways I think it's quite strange. I mean, when I think of myself at 10, I had much more responsibility.

Interviewer: What sort of things did you do?

Mother: Well, I mean, we would regularly go off to the cinema on Saturday afternoons, which was a bus ride away.

Jane: The shops. You went shopping with your friends.

Mother: We went shopping –

Interviewer: Was this in London?

Mother: No, it wasn't in London, no.

Jane: That's probably why. We live in London with lots of cars.

Mother: Yes, I – it was a different world.

Jane: Where you go [i.e. back to childhood home], there is only about one car every half hour. You went across the moors.

Mother: Yes, well, that's true. I could walk home from school without meeting a car. Very different world. So in some ways I find it quite strange, it's a very sheltered sort of existence [i.e. Jane's]. But on the other hand –

Jane: You do expect a bit more from me. You tell me off when I'm not being responsible enough. Otherwise you wouldn't tell me off.

Mother: Yes, this year, I think, now. Yes.

Interviewer: This year? Is that connected with the school year, do you mean? Or just this year because now she's 10?

Mother: I just – I don't know. It's just arrived at that sort of time. It just feels right – it's not to do with the school year or the age or anything.

Interviewer: Yes.

Mother: It's largely because Jane seems to want to do these things. And her friends are doing it. Which I think –

During this conversation, it emerged that when considering the question of how much responsibility Jane had or should have, her mother was balancing memories of her own childhood as a reference point, with her recognition of the differing – and more dangerous – environment within which Jane's childhood was being enacted. She also considered her daughter's agency as relevant, for, in explaining why she is letting Jane go to school with friends now, she brought into play a new factor: the concept of readiness; it seemed 'right' now that Jane should take more responsibility, and she backed up her argument – Jane's 'friends are doing it'. Indeed, mothers commonly consult each other about the next steps in handing over responsibility, and at Greenstreet some of the mothers, living in the same area, told me they had agreed together that they must now let their Year 5 children go to school alone or, preferably, with friends. Thus whilst in her own childhood, she suggested, she did not experience her own independent activity as a matter for parental question or worry, nowadays each step of the way towards use of the streets had to be the object of careful deliberation, taking a range of factors into account.

Jane herself demonstrated that she was familiar with her mother's stories of her childhood and with the scenes of that childhood. It emerged in this excerpt and elsewhere in the conversation that she fully understood the issues her mother was grappling with. The new freedom to go to school with her friends was achieved through consideration of a number of factors, including her mother's recollections. Like other children in these studies, Jane was more inclined to accept protection and commands which aimed at her physical welfare than with those aimed at socialization. For instance, in another conversation – this time with a friend at school – she claimed that she found it very boring when her mother insisted that she tidy her room; she preferred an untidy room 'where you climb about' above the littered objects. Her friend added that, though he knew why mothers 'went on' about tidy rooms – because you could hurt yourself on strewn objects – if it was your room, you had a right to keep it as you wished.[9]

Generational processes can be seen at work in these accounts by parents. The perceived cohort differences between their childhoods in the 1960s and 1970s and those of their children growing up in the 1990s form one basis for how parents thought about and shaped parent–child relations and their children's childhoods. Two main differences between childhoods past and present emerge in these accounts: external social conditions and parent–child relations. Environmental dangers necessitated stronger parental supervision than in the past, but off-setting these were the increased opportunities for children nowadays, such as sports facilities and clubs. Parents also identified democratization of parent–child relations as a general social trend, so that child respect for parents and parental discipline was giving way to more equal relationships, characterized by negotiation and compromise (cf. du Bois-Reymond *et al.* 1993). For some parents, this democratization was engineered through the increased knowledgeableness of children nowadays. As another mother commented:

> I don't know, the younger generation seems to be into, the kids nowadays – to me they're like 9 going on 19, and they want to know everything, they want to do everything, they know it all, they've done it, you can't talk to them. I didn't seem to have that problem when I was a child. I used to sort of [say], 'Yes, Mum' even if it was wrong. 'Yes, Mum', 'No, Mum', but, I don't know, it's the times that are changing, you've just got to go with the times as well.[10]

A further strand in parents' thinking was that the remembered character of their own childhoods had a bearing on what they should 'give' their children now; exploration and freedom to roam was to be replaced by structured, supervised outdoors experience and exercise, and by careful consideration of when and how far to 'let their children go'. In making these points, parents can be understood as making sense of how their past (remembered) experiences relate to the ways they try to influence their own children's lives. They are not just concerned for the quality of their children's lives; they are also managing their memories and linking these to an understanding of their own journey from the past to the present (cf. Giddens 1991: Ch. 3).[11]

Discussion

In considering the generationing processes whereby child–parent relationships are understood and within which childhoods are acted, I have drawn on parents' as well as children's accounts. A general issue is how far parents aim to reproduce or transform childhood. Clearly, childhood is understood by parents as a social status characterized by the need for protection, and by parental duty to supply it. Parents identify changes in how parental protection was understood in the past and is understood now. The notion of the safe outside world includes implicitly the idea that as a parent one can rely on good behaviour by other adults – they will not molest one's children. And furthermore, some explain that in the old days adults took collective responsibility for children's safety, and in the case of the account of a West Indian childhood, for disciplining children. In these accounts, it seems that people think they are doing parenting nowadays in a society which has privatized and individualized child-rearing.

This point links in with a 'risk society' set of conceptions; that nowadays people live in a society where many if not all aspects of life and decision-making involve taking risks, facing dangers. These ideas were expressed in parents' acceptance that traffic and strangers present dangers beyond their control; they have to protect their children and gradually expose them to using the outside environment (as Jane and her mother discussed). Even more risky is the education system. Parents in the Risk Study explained that secondary schools locally varied enormously in quality; it was up to individual children to do well enough at primary school (and primary schools offered varying qualities of education) to get into the better secondaries. Some wealthier parents were planning to pay for private education. Thus, again, children's experiences were at the mercy of an individualized set of forces, their own efforts and their parents' financial resources. Parents and children were making decisions on schools in a society which had not taken, or had shrugged off, responsibility for equality of school experience and of educational opportunity. Child–parent relationships have to be understood in these contexts. As I have briefly noted, some parents paid great attention to their children's homework; children themselves were aware that individual parental resources could determine their educational future (as Simon told me). Thus children and parents are tied together in their concerns.

The very close ties between children and parents described by the young people can be perhaps understood in part in the UK's privatized, individualized understanding of child–parent relationships. As the brief summaries I gave showed, these young people set out a precise and specific character for child–parent relations: identification of the family as the centrepiece of children's affections, their mother's central role as carer and confidante, negotiation within an overall framework of obedience, dependence and interdependence, participation within a framework of apprenticeship. As far as English childhoods are concerned, I think these characteristics belong to the present day and might not have been expressed, or expressed so clearly and forcibly by earlier generations of children. For instance, in the 1940s (to dredge up my own memories) when I was a child aged 9, traffic and strangers were not proposed as important dangers, we went to school unaccompanied by adults, and played outside after school; we thought the education system (though intrinsically divisive) divided people at age 11 not according to effort, but according to intelligence and we did not think we could do much about that; people did not question the quality of the secondary school. In sum, children in those old days, one might suggest, were not so tied physically, financially and emotionally to 'the family' or to parents; in important respects we were children of the welfare state. As against that, it is important and interesting that those people in my samples whose parents were born abroad, especially in the Indian subcontinent, expressed a closeness to family founded on duty and life-long responsibility, which is rooted in cultural and for some religious tradition.[12] Yet as I shall discuss in Chapter 5, these family values are somewhat in tension with the demands and opportunities of the education system and the job market. So perhaps it is arguable that the character of childhoods in England – or at any rate in London – may perhaps (we have no comparable evidence) have changed over the last 50 years (for discussion of current childhoods as crisis-ridden, see Chapters 7 and 9).

Running through this chapter, too, are allusions to cohort effects. At individual levels, children and parents negotiate their relationships in relation to childhoods lived in a changing society, to new ideas about child–parent relations, and to the development of a 'risk society'. More generally, we can see cohort effects at group levels. Parents who immigrate from differing cultures all watch over their children going through a specific education system in a strange society. Traffic and housing policies, mediated by parental response, have effects across the board on this cohort of children's daily lives.

Finally, I note that close ties between children and parents are described by young people across the age-range (5–13). Though the older ones talk of achieving greater independence, both girls and boys also talk of reciprocal affection, 'family times' and responsibilities to their families. Some UK studies of slightly older people – aged 16 (Brannen 1996), 15–19 (Allatt 1996), 16–18 (Ribbens MacCarthy 2001), and 11–16 (Langford et al. 2001) – confirm the proposition that the adult concept of a *Sturm und Drang*-laden 'adolescence' is in need of revision. Young people's accounts indicate, of course, variations, but central is young people's strong sense of connectedness with family life, with emphasis on personal responsibility and individual accountability, and with high valuation of parents' emotional support for them.

5 | Childhood work

This chapter continues the enterprise of studying how child–adult relations are constructed, maintained and modified. It progresses through a series of takes on work and education. First I look at the scholarization thesis, and consider children as workers. Then I take up twin running themes in the state UK education scene in order to consider their broad implications for the construction of childhoods: the pervasiveness of social class issues, and the suspicion of mothers. Third I draw on school life in two classrooms in order to chart how children's experiences and understandings of school-childness have changed in response to education policy changes. Fourth I look at some evidence on the activities of mothers and children in intersections between home and school.

Scholarization

Work and education: the scholarization of childhood

How do generational processes help us understand how childhood is understood? This chapter considers childhood in relation to education, since in western societies, including the UK, getting an education (at home and school) is regarded as the principal activity of childhood.

Qvortrup's scheme, shown in Figure 5.1, adapts a typology developed by Rogers and Standing (1981) for the majority world, where some of children's work may be paid – in family and non-family businesses – and some unpaid – at home and at school. It usefully draws attention to categories of children's work, including those which take place but are hidden from

Table 5.1 Children's work

	paid work	*unpaid work*
home	family work	daily duties
non-home	wage work	schoolwork

(*Source*: Qvortrup 1991: 20)

view in western industrialized countries. Children's work was one focus of enquiry in the Childhood as a Social Phenomenon project in 16 industrialized countries; participants were asked to document national data, and/or studies on work. In practice, they found detailed data on school activity, and some data on household work, but little on waged work and even less on 'family work'. As Qvortrup (1991: 25–32) comments, some of this lack reflects the illegal character of paid work by children, but the concentration in national data on school activity indicates its status as the proper activity of children. To the extent that only economically useful work is the basis for social esteem, the assumption that children do not work complements the low social esteem of childhood.

Qvortrup (1985) and Zelizer (1985) have described the processes whereby children have been excluded from the division of labour in western industrialized countries. Instead they have been positioned both ideologically and in practice in schools; childhood has been scholarized; the proper activities of children are as learners, not as workers; their relations with adults (nowadays parents and teachers) are those of dependency, just as they were when children worked in family workshops or factories. 'Children are now, as before, subjected to authority, dependent, dispossessed and without rights' (Qvortrup 1985: 139). But Qvortrup asks us to rethink childhood, to recognize it as a permanent social category, which contributes to the maintenance and advancement of the social order:

> Children take part in socially necessary activities, contribute towards the accumulation of knowledge and labour power to be used in society, are permanently a part of social renewal, and from an early age are an integral part of social organisation.
>
> (Qvortrup 1985: 142)

So there is a central conflict within adult understandings of modern, western, childhoods: scholarized and dependent or working contributors to the social order. The process of exclusion has also been justified and massively supported by the theorizing of psychologists, whose focus on child development and socialization was uncritically accepted by functionalist sociologists (Qvortrup 1985: 129–32; Prout and James 1990).

More recent studies on children and work

Until the mid-90s, in line with the designation of children as non-workers, there was little UK research on children's work, beyond the collection of numbers in paid work. A review of studies on children's work shows that between two-thirds and three-quarters of children do some paid work before the school-leaving age (16) (Mizen *et al.* 1999). Recent studies provide information about the work young people do and what work means to them.

Virginia Morrow (1994) studied the written accounts of out-of-school daily life by 730 young people aged 11 to 16. Of these, 40 per cent described doing some kind of domestic labour; 38 per cent did other labour (wage labour, marginal economic activity and non-domestic family labour); some did both domestic and other labour. Morrow here uncovers economically useful activity by children, whether paid or unpaid. She argues 'that we should move away from the sociological view of children as burdens who, as social actors, do little more than consume goods and services whether within their families or in the education system' (1994: 142). Children, she found, do paid work in order, variously, to buy consumer goods, to do something outside school, to feel confident and independent and more 'adult'. In these ways, we can argue, they are challenging childhood as proposed to them by participating in economic activities more commonly understood as limited to adults.

Vinod Chandra (2001) examined the meanings of the work young people (aged 10–16) do at home and in the family business – a corner shop, through discussions with 20 young people in Coventry (UK) and Lucknow (India). In terms of the typology quoted above, he studied an area between the paid and unpaid: the family business in which all members work unpaid and which provides the family income. He shows how all family members contribute to the 'family work order' which requires each person, according to strength and ability, to take responsibility for tasks at home and in the shop. Young people contribute, both through working in the shop and through domestic work, which frees up adults to work in the shop. This study shows that the traditional family enterprise of the pre-industrial society continues today – both in the UK and India.[1] Children and adults are engaged in a common enterprise to keep the family economically and socially afloat, and the young people value their contributions accordingly.[2] This study can be somewhat generalized to the more common UK situation, where adults do paid work outside the home; young people's domestic work both reduces adults' domestic work and frees up their energy for their paid work. Within the home, mothers welcome their children taking on self-care partly because it reduces their own childcare workload (Mayall 1994: Ch. 2).

Mizen *et al.*'s study (2001a) followed, over a year, 70 young people (aged 11–15) who worked for pay, and explored with them experiences of and feelings about work. They found that the principal motive for working was financial; young people wanted money for a range of childhood activities, including consumer spending. For some, having a source of income meant they could contribute directly to the household economy by taking pressure off parents; they bought their own clothes, shoes and school meals, and paid for leisure activities, or bought groceries for family consumption. Paid work meant they felt more independent and had more control over their daily life. Work experience was useful when considering their future work, and in demonstrating commitment and maturity to potential employers. (see also the papers in Mizen *et al.* 2001b).

These studies indicate that work, whether paid or unpaid, is an important feature of many young people's lives. In view of Qvortrup's scholarization thesis, I was interested in whether young people consider any of their activities come under the heading 'work'.

How do young people talk about work?

In my Childhood Study, Year Fives at North Primary School talked to me in pairs, and I encouraged them with a topic list to describe and reflect on the social positions of motherhood, fatherhood and childhood and on their daily lives (in all, 13 pairs plus one boy on his own). I did not introduce the topic 'work' but, if they mentioned it, encouraged exploration. Out of these 14 sessions, seven pairs made no mention of work in connection with children's lives in general or their own lives. Three described housework and childcare as work. One referred to homework without offering a definition. Three said school was work. Here are some examples.

These two made no mention of school as work, but said 'housework' and childcare lifted them temporarily out of the category 'child':

Interviewer: Do you think of yourself as a child, or as not a child sometimes?
Dominic: Sometimes when I do a proper job, carrying the shopping.
Elena: Sometimes when I do housework as well, cos my Mum has to look after the twins, that's when I don't feel really like a child. But I am a child, so.
Dominic: It's when you have to look after the kids [sometimes he cares for the children minded by his mother].

In the next example two girls discuss school as work. They introduced the apprenticeship theme – children get an education, but school is work of a lesser sort than adults'.

Interviewer:	What's it like being a child?
Jone:	It's good because you get a good education. And if you're good at some things and not at others you've got to try harder.
Interviewer:	So is being a child, getting an education?
Jone:	Sometimes, yes.
Nadia:	Well, I reckon adults is much harder than being a child, and the child part of your life is very, is enjoyable.
Interviewer:	More than being a grown up?
Both:	Yes [enthusiastic affirmations from both].
Nadia:	Because you don't have responsibility, like if you had children, not big responsibilities, like if they get hurt. And you don't have to go out to work, cos your work during the day is going to school.
Interviewer:	So do you think of school as work?
Jone:	Yes, because you do work, don't you?
Interviewer:	Yes, but I wondered, because you said it's not like going out to work.
Jone:	Yes, because adults do harder work.

Finally, two boys define work as something done for essential money; hence school is not really work.

Interviewer:	Are there some good things about being you at the moment?
Frank:	You don't have to work. You don't have to get money to live.
Interviewer:	You don't have to work?
Frank:	Well, you see, like, your dad and mum are the people who go to work, and you just go to school to learn and you don't exactly have to, like when you're an adult you have to do much harder work.
Interviewer:	Do you [Husain] agree with that?
Husain:	Mm.
Interviewer:	What about school, for instance? [Interviewer's leading question!]
Husain:	Well at school, you only go for like six and a half hours, but sometimes adults work for much longer than that.

The mixed messages coming across from these open-ended discussions interested me in directly pursuing the question of whether young people did regard work as part of their lives. So for fieldwork in the next school, North Secondary, I included a specific question about work: *What kinds of work do you do?* From 16 research conversations (14 with pairs and two with individuals), there were again mixed messages. In 13, young people replied to my question by referring to housework and of these two referred also to school. After a prompt (*What about school?*), six more defined school as work, in some cases hesitantly, and four did not. One pair vehemently disagreed with each other on the question. (In two cases, for various reasons the topic was not covered.) There were no perceptible differences by sex.

Some young people gave reasons why school was or was not work.

Interviewer: Apart from housework, do you do any other work?
[pause]
Interviewer: What about homework?
[laughter]
Interviewer: Is that work?
Leila: No, not really.
Jaya: Work is work round the house.
Leila: I don't think homework is work, because it's for you, not
             for someone else. Cleaning up is for everyone.

Another boy was adamant that school was not work, and said he was waiting for his thirteenth birthday, when he could (legally) get 'a paper round or something'. Another boy noted that work is what you get paid for. His friend (a girl) introduced a theme common to several: school is learning for the future. Another girl elaborated this apprenticeship point:

Roma: It's just part of life. It's not work because it's for me really,
            it's for me to learn, so I can get a job, so I can work when
            I'm older. It's like part of –
Interviewer: Whereas work is . . . ?
Roma: Like, earning money. School is just part of growing up.

Though school is not work, learning is a good thing in general, as two boys explained:

Isaac: So school is a very good thing. You don't know things, but
            you're learning some very good stuff. One day it's just like –
Thomas: It'll come in handy.
Isaac: Yes, like – boom! How did I know this? I just learned it at
            school!

So these north London young people present a complex picture as to the scholarization thesis. Work is that done to resource the family and, more generally, it is that which benefits others, especially the family. Whilst school activity can be described as work, it is much less hard than parents' work, and takes up less time. And for some, school activity is not work because it is for yourself, to learn what you need to know for future life, including a paid job. This perspective links back to one discussed in the previous chapter;

a common theme among young people is that childhood is, among other things, a privileged period with relatively few responsibilities, and a period where you can expect protection and provision, and should have free time. But they also engage in household tasks and childcare; some identify these as important contributions to the household; others, with fewer, lighter, shorter or less frequent tasks, see this as marginal activity. Thus it seems these young people do regard themselves as separated out from the world of serious, responsible work – that which is needed to resource families.[3]

As I noted in Chapter 4, the definitions of childhood absorbed by young people from their parents varied somewhat within broad commonalities. Adult expectations and cultural norms feed down into young people's thinking. Those whose parents had immigrated or who had close ties with other cultures were particularly strong on childhood as apprenticeship and on life-long family duty. They were expected to do routine household work as contribution to the family enterprise, to learn religious and cultural norms and to do well at school. It was much commoner for the East Year Fives to refer to school activity as work, which may reflect cultural norms that childhood comprises work, but also the sheer amount they had to get through in the formal classroom regime, and the fact that they (unlike the North Year Fives) had homework every night. The Year Eights in the two East seconday schools also conceptualized school activity as work; in their case a principal factor was probably not so much the school regime (much like that at North Secondary School), but parents' high expectations of their academic success (for gender issues on this see pp. 82–3).

By comparison with the young people in the three recent studies referred to earlier, the Childhood Study young people were slightly younger; most were below the legal age for paid work (13). Their lives were perhaps more closely bounded by home and school, by learning and living in those settings. Over-13s perhaps associate their activities more with adult work; they may see their activities as having economic significance, may be less absorbed by or committed to, or more disaffected from, school agendas. Perhaps the Childhood Study young people belonged more firmly in childhood, which they understood in contradistinction to adulthood.

Social class and maternal responsibility: issues in the provision of state education in the UK

Out of the range of issues integral to the provision of state education in England and Wales, I focus on two issues, social class and maternal responsibility, as key to understanding the social construction of childhood in the education system today.[4] Social class issues pervade the history and present of the system, interwoven with continuing debates over the appropriate division of responsibility for children's welfare and achievement, between the education providers and mothers, for whom a proxy term, these days, is often 'parents'. It was poor mothers, not wealthy ones, who were the concern of educationalists at the outset, and it still is today.

The process of the exclusion of all children from the workforce and their inclusion in school took place over a period when a substantial middle class was already in place, and they already used private schools for their children. The establishment of a state-funded education service was the site of intense debate from the mid-nineteenth century onwards (Hurt 1979). Evidently the children who were receiving little or no schooling were those of the poorer classes. Policymakers assumed that state education was to fit poorer people for their station in life. Wealthier parents would not use it on three main counts: they mostly did pay for their children's education already; they should pay for education; and they would not want their children to rub shoulders (literally) with the great unwashed. It is not by accident that this situation continues to this day. As George Walden (1996) forcefully expounds, in England and Wales, the reproduction of the polit-ical elite has been accomplished through the private education system; the 8 per cent of children who go to private schools belong to families who run the country, and who have no interest, literally, in ensuring that the 92 per cent get a good education. Rather they have an interest in reproducing, across the generations, their own power (in line with Bourdieu's argument).

> In no other European country do the moneyed and professional classes
> – lawyers, surgeons, businessmen, accountants, diplomats, newspaper
> and TV editors, judges, directors, archbishops, air chief marshals, senior
> academics, Tory ministers, artists, authors, top civil servants – in
> addition to the statistically insignificant but eye-catching cohort of
> aristocracy and royalty – reject the system of education used by the
> overwhelming majority pretty well out of hand, as an inferior product.
>
> (Walden 1996: 19)

The establishment of schooling for the poor exposed a second issue which has dogged education ever since: the appropriate division of responsibility between the state and mothers for the welfare of children. For, once these poorest children were made visible in school, they were seen to be both hungry and subject to infectious diseases. Money spent on education services would be wasted unless they were fed and medically treated. Subsequent debates among the ruling classes around child ill-health and the scandal of high rates of child mortality focused on competing causes: maternal neglig-ence or maternal poverty (Gordon *et al.* 1991: 128; Harris 1995: Ch. 3). A key figure was Sir George Newman, appointed as first Medical Officer at the Board of Education in 1907, whose annual reports considered the evid-ence; for instance, his 1916 report on child mortality pointed to both poverty and maternal fecklessness and ignorance (Mayall 1981: Ch. 1). Remedies through state action (school meals, medical inspection and treatment) were embarked on only slowly and grudgingly, since such remedies might indicate that the state was taking on parental responsibilities and thereby further weaken maternal sense of responsibility (Hurt 1979: Chs 5, 6). Concern for the health status of the nation's soldiery was one impetus for such interventions; the child as national investment was emerging (Hendrick 1994: 14).

As is well known, the private and state divide in the education system in England and Wales persists to this day; the state system has been in the political hands, largely, of people whose own children do not use it (Adonis and Pollard 1997). The private system is insulated from the state system but structures its character; this divide accounts for large classes, decaying buildings, teachers' low status and victim-blaming. Politicians may claim that they are keen to invest in the nation's children; but over the last 20 years the measures adopted by both Conservative and Labour parties have been hostile, focusing as they do on identifying failure by 'testing children to destruction' (*Guardian*, 4 August 2000) rather than enabling them to learn.

Thus the state education system has been marked by low funding, as befits inferior children, and by suspicion of all those involved: the children, the teachers, the local education authorities, the mothers. Distinctive in the history of education in England and Wales is the long sequence of studies into links between 'home background' and school achievement (Ouston and Hood 2000: Ch. 2).[5] The 1960s emphasis (CACE 1967: Ch. 2) on the home as the main site of early education, led on to policy moves to 'involve' 'parents' with school agendas, but both trends allowed for some homes being problematized.

The power of history to structure present-day policies provides a context for the next two sections: on childhood experience at school, and on intersections between home and school.

Schools as sites of agency and learning

School sites for experience

The enduring, persistent relations between ideologies underpinning state education and provision on the ground can be seen in the physical conditions of our schools. I flag up here, briefly, three topics: numbers of children, buildings and outside space, and health-care.

Over the 1980s and 1990s, *numbers of children* per school increased and teacher–child ratios worsened (*Guardian*, 3 October 1995). Thus the number of infant classes with over 30 children rose to a peak of 485,000 in 1998; a determined drive downwards by the Labour government reduced such classes to 30,000 (*Guardian Education*, 7 November 2000: 2–3). Crowded schools lead to more accidents and stress. Large classes mean more pressure on space, decreased access by children to teachers, and teacher difficulties in looking after children and helping them learn. Current research is showing that children in smaller classes are doing better on literacy and numeracy work, and this is especially noticeable among the 25 per cent 'weakest attainers' (*Guardian Education*, 7 November 2000: 2–3).

During the Conservative era (1979–97) spending on *school buildings* fell and the current Labour government is faced with the consequences of many years of neglect. Our CHIPS survey (in 1993–4) showed that on a number of indicators the physical environment – buildings, playspace and playground equipment – was reportedly poor in nearly half of schools surveyed. Unsurprisingly, on average, the oldest buildings were poorest (Mayall *et al.* 1996: 244–5). Of particular concern to our respondents was the state of the lavatories, and the inadequacies of playground equipment. According to Simon (1988: 26), Keith Joseph (Minister for Education 1981–6) argued that excellent education could take place in 'crummy' buildings (was he thinking of Harrow, his alma mater?) but Joseph's point does not meet the objection that market forces are acceptable where people pay for private education but that state provision should provide reasonable standards.[6]

Third, I consider *health-care*. At school, teachers stand in common law *in loco parentis* to the children (Stock 1994: Ch. 1). While health and safety legislation clearly covers employees, if teachers care for the children like the average careful parent, their legal duty is discharged. Traditionally, schools have relied on the add-on character of women's work; they will add caring on to their formal remit (see p. 16). The school health service (SHS) makes marginal impact on child health-care, being mainly for defect-spotting and referral (Mayall and Storey 1998). Our CHIPS data show that the informal health-care system, if it ever worked well, is breaking down under the impact of education policies, which have piled work onto women in schools. It is not surprising that mothers think the system fails children (Mayall 1994: Chs 5, 6) and CHIPS teachers confirmed their view. A House of Commons committee (1997, para. 87) argued (like us) that an SHS should provide hands-on care for children, and they noted (with unsurprising surprise) that there is 'a considerable degree of confusion about whose responsibility it should be to provide care for children with clinical needs at school' (para. 88). As far as I know, no steps have been taken to tackle this problem.

Schools are finding it difficult to carry out this 'add-on' work, to look after children when they are ill. Indeed mothers are being summoned to school to resume their childcare responsibilities; education policy ignores the incompatibility of expecting mothers both to do paid work and to care for their children.[7] Teachers and other staff are also finding that their classes contain more children requiring health-care.[8] Causes include the survival of children with chronic conditions (Heussler *et al.* 2000), inclusive policies and larger class sizes. Yet at the same time schools report cutbacks in the SHS and in specialist services to help them care for children (Mayall *et al.* 1996: Ch. 7; see also Polnay 1998).[9]

I give next some information about one of our CHIPS case-study schools, in order to explore the impact of education policies on children's experience. Town School (Mayall *et al.* 1996: 147–60), with 339 children (aged 5–11), was sited on an estate in a midlands town, and had a main building dating from the 1960s. In recent years, staff and children told us, the physical and social environment had worsened. The classrooms had been designed for no more than 24 children each; now they had 30 or more children each, and were cramped and uncomfortable for children and teachers. In order to accommodate more children, three new blocks, each with two classrooms and its own toilets, had been built in the playground, plus a separate toilet block. This not only meant reduced playspace; it meant poor sightlines, sharp corners – and more accidents. Staff thought they should supervise children's outside play, but there were not enough staff to monitor all spaces; so, as the children told us, often they were not allowed to play in some spaces – hence more crowding. In general, teachers thought that children had to be overcontrolled both in class and outside, and since curriculum times designated for physical exercise had been reduced in order to focus on core topics in the National Curriculum, they thought the school day was bad for children's health.

Here is the Year 5 teacher at Town School, whose class had 34 children, talking about children's school experiences:[10]

> *Year 5 teacher*: A lot of them, particularly the older boys, you know, feel that they are being kept in, they are being so tightly controlled, you've got to control them tightly because if you don't your classroom discipline ... And in effect the way every child in the classroom learns is affected. So it is a balance. I mean, I would think some children find it quite a strain, because they want to be, again particularly boys, older boys, they want to be out doing all these boyish things, they want to be running and climbing and jumping and they're not, they're kept down in the classroom ... their natural spirits are thwarted ... Because by their nature they want to be out, say doing PE activities all of the time and obviously they can't because they've got to be in the classroom learning. [The interviewer asked if the school was able to care for the children.] I mean, I think that perhaps

we ought to have it higher on our agenda than perhaps we have. But then when we're looking at all of the educational things that we've got to cope with for the children and all of the changes that have taken place, all the policies and the schemes of work and everything we've had to develop for each curriculum area, they have really taken over and things are getting, the pace of change has been very quick and what we're expected to be able to do in the classroom has also, is much more rigorous, so we're all very concerned about that, but I think underlying, realizing that the health and care of the child is important . . .

Interviewer: Are there any changes you would like to see?

Year 5 teacher: Well, it would possibly be nice to offer children the opportunity, particularly as they get older and more responsible for themselves, the opportunity to speak to somebody, just quietly and calmly ask them you know, are there any areas that you are concerned about, that you would like to talk with somebody about – and that could be a welfare assistant, ultimately it could be anybody that the child had chosen within the school, the person that the child feels happiest with, talking to and sharing their worries and concerns. I mean, I'm sure we don't do enough of that . . . I think it is the mental and emotional and psychological that is becoming more and more important. And I think that is becoming more important in how children learn and how they respond to education, because a lot of them are becoming very, one might call, sulky children, very sulky, very selfish, but it's because of these things that go on in their minds that they've got to cope with [later, like the school nurse, he refers to problems at home]. And school is probably an added pressure and therefore this is the cause of behavioural problems.

Under Local Management of Schools (LMS), the school had appointed a bursar – who occupied the former sick room, so now there was no designated space to care for children.[11] The school nurse explained that she was covering 22 schools in a 30 hour week, over a 'large geographical area'; that she visited this school only two or three times a term; and that her work with the children took place 'in all sorts of nooks and crannies', where there was no privacy for children to 'open up to you, maybe about some worries they've got and they feel that they can't talk to either their parents or their class teacher'. She thought pressure on teachers to implement the National Curriculum was leading them (in some schools) to devalue children's health and downgrade links between health and education. It was sometimes up to her to say: 'Well, if you haven't got a healthy child or a child which is to its maximum potential in health, then their education is going to be restricted anyway, and I think the Head feels that, and does see that.'

Children's school experiences, and those of the adults (mainly women) at school, are structured by generational and gendered understandings. In the state system, these underpin low investment in schools. By long tradition, the eyes of the policymakers are on the future economic contribution children may make as adults. In complement, the focus is on the cognitive, with little attention to links between the bodily and the cognitive (Bendelow and Mayall 2000). *Mens sana in corpore sano* applies only in the private sector (where they have 'matrons'). Women staff in state schools are expected to 'cope', in whatever conditions, and so are the children's mothers.

Experiencing school in the 1990s

In this section I consider the formal and informal school regime in relation to children's experiences of school, in two classes, in the 1990s.[12] The aim is to interrelate education policy changes with processes of change in children's experiences during the 1990s. To what extent have persistent relations between the social group children and the social group teachers been modified? Have children's school experiences changed? How do they characterize their school activity?

The 1990s have seen great changes in state education policy, particularly on primary education. From the time of data-collection in the first study (1990–1) to the fourth (1997–8) initiatives include: implementation of a national curriculum, national tests, frequent inspection and competition between schools. Nowadays, children work to the National Curriculum. Government guidelines emphasize a literacy and numeracy session each day and science as the third key subject. Arts and sports are pushed to the sidelines (Pollard *et al.* 1994: 112–18; Richards 1998). Since what is to be learned in each subject is prescribed, schools have moved from an integrated, sometimes topic-based approach, to the division of the day into formal subjects. Testing has become commonplace and overt – on spellings, times-tables, mental arithmetic, the 'facts' of history and geography. National tests take place in Year 2 (Key Stage 1) and Year 6 (Key Stage 2), when children are 7 and 10.

In complement to these changes in educational policy, formal child–teacher relationships have changed. In order to expose each child to the knowledge they are meant to acquire, covering a wide range within each 'subject', teachers are adopting whole-class methods (which are also favoured by the inspectorate), whereby they tell the children what they have to know and help each child absorb the knowledge by taking notes, reading the relevant material, revising the topic. In order for this method to work, children have to be quiet, docile and concentrated on the teacher's agenda; the teacher has to maintain order and promote herself as the person with the appropriate knowledge (see also Pollard *et al.* 1994; Campbell 1998).

In response to the same policies, homes have also changed as sites of child–parent relationships. Children's worries about their test performances may spill over into relationships at home. Children and parents are encouraged by political rhetoric to think that school achievement is a matter of individual responsibility and that high achievement will lead to good jobs and a secure future. Since the time of my studies, there are further demands on parents, who, from the late 1990s, are increasingly urged by political initiatives to work with their children on homework tasks.

Greenstreet Primary School (1990–1)
The Year Fives I worked with at Greenstreet were among the last cohorts to escape national testing at age 7 and 10.[13] School-based tests in Year 6, as well as parental and child preference, were the basis of decisions about secondary school, Year 6 was commonly regarded as somewhat stressful, while these processes were taking place. There was little pressure downwards to Year 5.

Year Fives spent their school day (8.50–3.30) mainly seated in groups of four or five around tables in the classroom; they chose whom to sit with, and thus maintained their friendship groups in class (though sometimes the teacher moved a child who chatted too much and worked too little). On three days, the day started with a whole-school assembly; on two days the class gathered together to bring news from home ('news-time'). There was a 15-minute morning break-time and a lunch break of 70 minutes. After lunch there was a daily quiet half-hour after lunch when the children read a book of their own choice, and for the last half-hour, the teacher read to the children from a storybook. There was homework once a week – to be done at the weekend.

The children each worked at their own pace on the basics of literacy and numeracy, working their way through course books. They helped each other with this work. They also worked collaboratively on projects. For instance, during one term they studied the geography, history and culture of China, and during the next focused on health promotion; groups researched and wrote up subtopics within these projects. Most days the teacher did some whole-class teaching, mainly to start them off with tasks, and thereafter acted as facilitator. The classroom was noisy, with periodic (and increasingly angry) requests by the teacher to reduce noise levels. The children each kept a running list of tasks to be accomplished, and though some complained because the list never ended, they chose at what pace to work, and how much of each task to get through. Outside school hours, the children were free of school-related commitments, except for a home-work task (up to one hour) at the weekend.

East Primary School (1997–8)
At East, the day also lasted six-and-a half hours, with a morning and lunch break. The Year Fives followed the National Curriculum. They had done the Key Stage 1 tests at age 7, and the year's work in Year 5 was overtly planned to prepare them for Key Stage 2 tests in Year 6. There was a clearly set out timetable, allocating time for each subject; the morning was taken up with a literacy session and then a numeracy session. The predomin-ant method in each session was whole-class teaching, followed by indi-vidual work. The children sat at tables in groups of four to six; for literacy and numeracy sessions, the teacher grouped them by ability, and, like the Greenstreet children, they worked through course books at their own pace; the teacher worked mainly with the least able. In the afternoon, the chil-dren chose whom to sit with. They worked hard all day, and conversation was muted. The teacher set homework every night, usually in the form of learning and revision of the day's sessions.

An extra edge to the East regime was provided by the fact that the vast majority of the children came from families where the parents had immi-grated from the Indian subcontinent and were, I gathered from the chil-dren, struggling financially to make their way. School staff were overtly committed to giving these children the best possible start in the competitive education system. In turn the children brought to school habits of obedi-ence, respect for their elders, and commitment to a future in which they would help their families.

What the children said about school
In 1990–1 Greenstreet maintained remnants of 'progressive' education ideologies; to some extent children's own knowledge and active learning were valued. They brought news from home, read books chosen by them-selves, participated in group work and project work. In 1997–8 at East, under the influence of government policy changes, children were the objects of adult work; they were to learn what the teacher told them, in line with national guidelines.

However, in common amongst all these 9-year-olds is the clear under-standing that school is controlled by adults, whom children must obey; and learning literacy and numeracy is essential for later stages of education and for getting a job (understandings shared by children across a range of studies and across time; e.g. Cullingford 1991: Ch. 6; Mayall *et al.* 1996;

Edwards 2000). At this point, the two sets of accounts diverge. Greenstreet children did not report personal stress to achieve; it was enough if they conformed and did what they were told. There was a laid-back feel to the children's accounts, which complemented the relatively easy-going regime directed by the teacher. East children, by contrast, expressed an individual responsibility and burden to learn what they needed to know; they told me that their teacher continually stressed that the work was preparation for the Year 6 tests, which in turn would determine which secondary school they would go on to. Their accounts complemented the adult-designed ethos represented by hard work, testing, and competition. Their accounts also fitted with the interdependent responsibility they had been taught towards their families, now and in the future.

The children's accounts of child–teacher relations also related to the specific character of the two teacher-led regimes. At Greenstreet, where working with and talking with friends was accepted ideologically, relations were sometimes fraught, for, as the teacher said, she found the noise levels irritating and, as the children said, was 'always' shouting at them and nagging them. Furthermore, because she perceived her task as to initiate and encourage children's activity in learning, in a mixed ability class, she thought she should explain the tasks in detail. Most of the children felt they spent far too much time sitting around being given instructions: '[It's really boring] when the teacher keeps on talking and she keeps on telling you over and over again and she doesn't let you go and get on with it' (cf. Cullingford 1991: Ch. 8).

The children stressed that what they really enjoyed was doing things and achieving things, but for much of the time the work was repetitive (writing up 'in best') and 'boring' (compare Christensen and James 2001). The best bits of the day were where they were active and agentic: the silent reading time, working on the computer, PE and games, and any activity where they gained a sense of achievement. One boy's summary of school experience speaks for many children:

> School is boring. It lasts six whole hours and 30 whole minutes. From 10 to 9 till 3.30. When I walk in the school gate at 10 to 9 I feel tired. When I walk out of the gate at 3.30 I feel happy. I think the most important people in school are children. The best part of the day is when we go home.

By comparison the East children recounted distinctive experiences of child–teacher relations. They said their teacher was strict and made them work hard all day. But they respected him as having the knowledge they needed in order to accomplish this year's work, and to prepare them for the Year 6 tests. They did not comment on his personal attributes and failings (as Greenstreet children did). Their stance reflected the regime he implemented in order to work with the National Curriculum. He was a very experienced teacher, and ran a very orderly and quiet classroom; he had established an atmosphere of purposeful work as the norm. The children certainly thought they were expected to work hard, and most did, though a few, less committed and less conformist, were quietly reproved from time to time.

The young people's accounts also indicate changes in interrelations between school and home. Clearly, home and mothers' work are structured around school demands (Smith 1988: Ch. 5; David *et al.* 1993; Vincent and Warren 2000). Greenstreet mothers described how they managed the home partly to meet these demands – that children be there on time, that they be rested, clean, washed, fed, appropriately dressed, with equipment needed for the day. And children too noted that getting to school was demanding and often stressful. But apart from these demands, children's accounts of home life in 1991 suggested a domain separate from the school and much freer; activity there included self-care and some minor housework, participation in the construction and maintenance of relationships, and enough free time for friends, play, TV and computers.

By the end of the 1990s, schools were impacting more strongly than before on life at home (Hood 1999). The East School children in 1997–8 had homework each day, mainly revision and learning, and some complained that it took up to two hours. Homework demanded by school competed with the home's cultural norms – attendance at mosque and housework duties.[14] Out-of-school sports, language and arts activities had to compensate for poor provision at school, squeezed out by government policies. The domains of school and home both carried adult expectations that children were workers; expectations that they endorsed. Life at home, therefore, offered very little 'free time' – which the children valued highly.

The intermediate domain: intersections between home and school in the lives of mothers and children

In this section, I consider mothers' and children's activities across the home and school. For, whilst it is appropriate to understand children as objects of the education system – a positioning exacerbated by recent policies on home–school agreements and homework (see below), yet it is also appropriate to consider children, as well as mothers, as agentic contributors to negotiations in an intermediate domain between home and school.

The recent history of home–school relations in the UK continues to emphasize early twentieth-century themes. Mothers, not fathers, are the target of moves to improve home–school relationships, but this is covert in policy moves. Social policies continue to position mothers as the parents who are responsible for childcare, policies which are rooted in UK psychological literature (Walkerdine and Lucey 1989: Chs 1–3). The relations of ruling, wilfully blind to the contradictions in its policies, exhort mothers, especially lone mothers, to go out to work, regard them as responsible for childcare and do not provide adequate daycare services; children are defined as not competent to be at home 'alone' (Standing 1999a). The scene outside any primary school any day is commonplace confirmation of these points; overwhelmingly it is mothers who take and pick up, and go in to talk to the teacher. But they are a 'silent majority' (Reay 1995) – taking the blame but not getting the credit, assigned responsibility without authority in patriarchal structures (Ribbens 1993a; MacLachlan 1996).

Recent policy moves have renewed the issue of mothers' participation in education. Here I consider the Home–School Agreement (HSA), homework policies, and intersections of gender and generation in the workings through of these policies.

The Home–School Agreement (HSA)

All state schools in England and Wales were required to have an HSA in place by September 1999; this is proposed as helping to tie homes and schools more closely together in a partnership towards children's educational achievement. A study of implementation (Ouston and Hood 2000) using a postal questionnaire and four case studies found that, in accordance with DfEE guidelines, almost all schools were consulting (more or less fully) with parents, but of those with an HSA in place in September 1999 only 30 per cent consulted students, and of those still working on it, only 40 per cent did so. Among other things, the questionnaire and case studies asked for perceived advantages and disadvantages in HSAs. The general point, made by teachers, governors, parents and students, was that those people who are working well together will continue to do so, but those who are not will not. The HSA initiative conceptualizes the key relations as those between the adults concerned, through which they will cooperate on school agendas (Ouston and Hood 2000: 9) but the concept of partnership between parents and teachers is challenged by the content and underlying assumptions of the agreements:

> It is a curious definition of partnership when the school's commitments appear to be what they should be doing anyway as part of their daily work, while parents and students are instructed as to their behaviour.
> (Ouston and Hood 2000: 75)

They note that parents and students have little scope for making their wishes and expectations met. Within the HSA, as traditionally, good parents support the school's work, problem parents are unsupportive and make difficulties for the school. Students are expected to comply with school rules and agendas (as they would be anyway).

It may be that the HSA will fade away, or simply become a statement of school rules and ethos, available to parents and students as part of schools' publicity brochures. But this piece of current government policy plays a part in the processes whereby childhood is constructed.

It seems that the HSA proposes childhood achievement as partly a function of parental behaviour and collaboration with the school; and as ever 'parental' is proxy for 'maternal'. In DfEE and school discourses, the agency of children themselves is downplayed. In practice, schools vary in their respect for children's participation rights (see Chapter 6: 99).[15]

Homework

Whether or not homework is any use to children's learning is a contested point (Cowan *et al.* 1998), but the present government adopts a 'commonsense' approach: it is obviously good, and should start at 5 years (Smith 2000). Currently, homework schemes have been developed both nationally and locally to 'transform the home setting into an educational context' (Edwards and Alldred 2000: 437), by asking 'parents' to work with their children on assignments. In 1998, the DfEE issued detailed guidelines on the government's expectations on the form, content and duration of homework for different age-groups (DfEE 1998; Smith 2000).

Homework also raises the questions whether it affects relations within the family and home–school relations and whether children are agents in their own education. Recent studies throw light on these issues.

From mothers' perspectives, homework puts additional stress on time-use. Time after school now has to include homework as well as afterschool clubs, leisure, eating, television and storytimes (Ribbens 1994: 114–17). Mothers (in New Zealand) report a range of relational experiences, from harmonious to acrimonious (Cowan *et al.* 1998).

A study with young people aged 9–14 found they played 'an active part in their parents' involvement in their education both in the home and at school . . . some by initiating, facilitating or going along' with it; others by 'discouraging or resisting' it (Edwards 2000: 1; Alldred *et al.* 2002). An important issue for young people was the privacy of their home lives, and their wish to maintain control over how much the school knew about these. They also, importantly, thought that home was a place for relaxing, doing what you choose, while school is about rules and timetables. Many did not wish the home to become affected by school agendas.

In my own three-generational family, in brief, I observe that:

- the school assumes the child will take home the assignment and give it to her mother – thus the child as agent must act to position herself as the child as object of the teacher/mother surveillance system;

- homework assignments are designed on the basis that 'parent' and child will work together on them; and therefore homework will have to be carried out in the distracting environment of the mother's workplace – the kitchen/living room;[16]
- children's anger at incursions into their free time and resentment that their mother is behaving like a schoolteacher – for the school – intersects with their mother's annoyance at the assumption that she will work with the children on school matters;
- everyone's time at home is pressurized;
- and more broadly, homework is divisive: it favours those children who come from well resourced families (maternal time and knowledge, books, computers).

We can use Margaret Archer's account of relational processes (1998: 82–4; and see pages 34–5) to consider my daughter's responses to homework. She, faced with school demands and her children's highly charged resistance to homework, took action. She told her children that homework was an undesirable but required feature of home-life, settled the children down once a week to polish it off (on a Thursday, thus leaving the weekend free), and rewarded them and herself with a supper of everyone's favourite foods. We see here, in little, processes across time, whereby people transform a structure (a policy) through their agency, into a workable practice.[17]

Two case studies

Here I take two detailed cases to consider the case for children alongside mothers as workers in the intermediate domain.

Girls and their migrant mothers

In the Childhood Study, I learned that where parents had immigrated from other societies, they and their children continuously negotiated with the demands and possibilities of the education system, while reproducing or modifying their cultural traditions. They were 'actively engaging with their cultural frameworks, while continuously transforming them' (Bhachu 1993: 101). Education in the UK is a key topic for consideration as regards girls, since high educational levels are beneficial to the family, but require modifications in lifestyle during the process of acquiring them.[18] Thus an educated girl brings honour to the family; she may enter a profession and bring much-needed money into the family; she may marry better than an uneducated girl (Gavron 1997: Ch. 3).

Of particular interest is how Muslim girls and their mothers negotiated attention to the (somewhat conflicting) demands of school and home, within an overall patriarchal moral framework (cf. Husain and O'Brien 1998). As some of 'my' Year 8 girls explained, doing well at school meant that some normal activities and duties had to give way, such as socializing with the (extended) family, and doing housework. Whilst, it seems, mothers expected to monitor closely every detail of their daughter's activities, including their homework, the girls brought into the home more exact knowledge of what the assignments entailed and of deadlines for delivery. To some extent they challenged their mothers' authority through this knowledge. Furthermore, whilst mothers, and to a lesser extent fathers, were already discussing what job their daughters should work towards, the girls again could contribute more realistic and appropriate knowledge to such discussions. Some of these girls also told me of a covert agenda, not discussed with parents; if they stayed at school to do A levels, and thence could propose going to university, they delayed marriage (see also Gavron 1997: Chs 3, 8).

This picture of mothers' desire for intense involvement in girls' activities was not evident in boys' accounts, though boys too were expected to achieve highly. How they spent their time was more up to them; it included less housework (though some) and regular time out at clubs and with friends. In their accounts there was little evidence of stressful supervision or of tension between expectations and worries. Since the girls' lives were lived entirely within the family (apart from school time) their relationships with their mothers were intense; their identities were shaped in interaction with their mothers' understandings of how women's lives should and could be lived, in relation to broader social understandings of gender roles in their Muslim communities. As Alibhai-Brown (2000: Ch. 7) discusses, immigration often makes more of an impact on women's thinking than on men's, essentially because as mothers they have to come to terms with their children's day-to-day experiences in schools, they place hopes on their children and have to help them through childhood and into adulthood in an unfamiliar and often hostile society.

These Year 8 girls were expounding processes in their working partnership with their mothers, where each brought to bear knowledge and experience to forge a workable way forward. The education system here provides a forum for mediating the public world of UK society with the private world of the family and its culture and heritage. Girls and mothers work through issues in the reproduction and transformation of women's lives, through their engagement with education, religion and economic demands.

Stuart and his mother
This 12-year-old told me he lived with his mother and stepfather; his father had a new family elsewhere, but Stuart maintained contact.[19] He explained he was responsible for doing well at school and getting a good job, since his father's maintenance contributions would stop once he left school. He told me he was blind in one eye (this was not obvious to the onlooker) but at

primary school he had told no one this (except his best friend) and he was isolated and bullied. His mother had written letters and asked the education authority for help, but this was slow in coming. His mother then engaged in negotiations with the secondary school to get his disability recognized, accepted and helped with. When he started secondary school, the class teacher made a point of encouraging the young people to talk about their disabilities in a whole-class session, and for Stuart this meant that his class-mates, armed with knowledge of his disability, became helpful, encouraging and friendly to him.

So Stuart took part in the negotiations between home and school, whereby his blindness was recognized and responded to. At home he and his mother worked together on his homework, including extra homework to help him catch up on literacy. Recently, too, they jointly made a cake and took it up to the school for his class to enjoy.

> *Interviewer*: What are the best things about life at home at present?
> *Stuart*: I'm doing fine. I'm doing more things around the house than I used to do. Like I can read words on the box [cake mix], and me and my Mum baked a cake for the school, and I could read the ingredients, and my Mum helped me and we made a cake and brought it to school –
> *Interviewer*: Was there a celebration at school?
> *Stuart*: No, it was my birthday, and cos my Mum couldn't run quickly to the shop and get a cake, we made one. [Discussion on the date of his birthday.] Because my Mum said, because I never had many friends, we never had a big party. But because now I have lots of friends, she's going to hire a hall and have big party.
> *Interviewer*: Is she proud of you now?
> *Stuart*: Yes, she's quite proud of me, because I've got friends and I'm settling in well.

His new friends, too, helped him negotiate between school demands and home life:

> They invite me to their house and help me do my homework. Bruce, I stayed at his house and I couldn't understand the homework, so he sits down with me and we do it together.

Stuart's story shows the processes he identifies whereby he and his mother acted at the start of his secondary school career to ensure the school did not repeat the mistakes of the primary school (cf. Ribbens 1993b). He thought their actions, with the cooperation of the teacher led to an improvement in his relations with his classmates and to his ability to work and achieve.

Stuart could now work at his schoolwork at home and school, with help from adults and friends in both; he noted again and again how pleased he was to be doing well with schoolwork and how happy he was to have friends now. His mother's actions to obtain help for her son at school were augmented by their joint actions to involve the school in his birthday, and to cement his friendships with his classmates by bringing a celebratory cake into the school.

This boy's experience at primary and secondary school, like the Town School's teacher and nurse earlier, highlights the pastoral function of schools, its benefits to children and the serious consequences of neglecting it. Clearly, as the Town staff indicated, all children should be respected as people, and given the chance to seek help, but for some children such opportunities are crucial, for instance those disabled by school agendas (see Alderson and Goody 1998 on integrated schools; Rutter 1994 on refugees; Kiddle 1998 on traveller children).

Concluding points

This chapter has explored the notion of children as workers, in the context of the power of history, across the generations. The class-based structure of the education system still implies underfunding of the state system and devaluing of the children who use it. State schoolchildren's work is not valued as such, in itself, by educators, but constantly viewed as suspect and needing to be tested; its value is future-oriented. Recent policies indicate that their mothers are still suspect, and must be marshalled into line. But evidence indicates that teachers' traditional concern for the whole child and for democratizing initiatives sometimes survives into the more top-down job they now find themselves doing (see Chapter 6: 99–101).

The data amassed in various studies indicate it is high time to reconsider 'work' and children's participation in it, in line with the typology on page 64. The notion that 'work' means direct, immediate economic contribution to society needs to be extended, as women have long argued, to include people work at home and in the intermediate and public domains. Clearly, many under-18s do paid work, and they also participate directly in the economic survival of the household, both by housework and by releasing parental time for paid work. Furthermore, like women, they engage in people work at home – and at school (see p. 11). And their activity at school, and for school at home, must be regarded as work since it contributes to the economy in the longer term. As I have also suggested, what they do at school, under the impact of education 'reforms' in the 1990s, looks more and more like work by any criteria; national policies redefine education as schooling for future employment.[20]

But the structuring of childhood is not solely carried out by the adults who legislate, deliver services and manipulate their lives. Young people themselves participate in structuring their childhoods and their futures. This is evidenced in their reflections on childhood, in their hard work at and for school, in their participation in family life, their interventions on 'parental involvement' and their discussions about their futures. I follow Margaret Stacey in suggesting the intermediate domain as a useful concept – bridging the private and public, and extend her argument to suggest that not only mothers, but children engage with professionals, directly and indirectly, to negotiate the quality of their lives.

Generationing and gendering processes have been explored to show how relationships between motherhood and childhood have been redefined through education policies in the 1990s (such as the HSA and homework policy). Thus mothers are now educators for the school, and children are schoolworkers at home. Children find themselves ever more scholarized, positioned under the joint surveillance of teachers and mothers, with free time reduced both in and out of school. I have suggested that these redefining processes are mediated by migration factors, since education has specific significance for those considering its intersections with their own cultures, and the importance of education as a means to improving family income.[21] In division of labour terms, the redistribution of responsibility for education away from schools and towards 'parents', exemplified through recent policies, seems likely to increase inequalities in educational opportunities.

We may finally want to say that education policy, along with other large-scale forces, is producing a new generation of children, with distinctive orientations to work and their futures. This point will be explored later, especially in Chapters 7 and 9.

| The moral status of childhood

In the previous two chapters I have explored processes in child–adult relations, mainly with parents and teachers. In this chapter, I want to take a specific topic within child–adult relations: processes whereby children's moral agency is or is not recognized and respected. It is partly because recent studies have made a point of listening to children, that we adults are learning what a burning issue their moral agency is for children. They occupy a moral space where adults do not always respect their moral agency but nevertheless expect them to take on responsibility, and in their daily interactions they encounter and grapple with moral dilemmas. There is a fault line between their experience and adult expectations of them.

I aim here to consider the relational processes whereby childhood is assigned certain characteristics by adults, and whereby those defined as adults and as children interact to reproduce and/or modify the acceptance and enaction of those characteristics. I start by considering children's moral agency, and then use young people's accounts to demonstrate the complexity of their engagement with moral issues. Then I go on to consider intersections of social and material contexts with the moral status of childhood: school, neighbourhood and home. Finally I discuss what kinds of explanations may be useful for better understanding of their moral status.

Children as moral agents

The idea of 'the child' as moral agent is one we (we adults in the UK) have been taught to find difficult, even a contradiction in terms. The dominant discipline providing knowledge about childhood – developmental psychology

– has proposed childhood as a series of stages, linked to age, with each successive stage bearing distinctive cognitive features, and children cannot proceed from one stage to the next until their cognitive abilities are sufficiently developed to appreciate the greater complexity of the next stage. Both Piaget and Kohlberg provide elaborate schemas showing these developments. Though adults who live with children are daily confronted by their moral agency and their lively discussions of moral issues, these adult experiences and these child activities do not form part of the common culture of UK understanding about children. Gareth Matthews (a US philosopher) suggests that 'the *idea* of developmental psychology has had a greater influence on the way adults think about children than have any specific findings of developmental psychologists, or any specific theories as to how children develop.' Adults generally, he argues, accept the idea that children go through various stages, and that the changes from stage to stage are changes 'from relative inadequacy to relative adequacy' (Matthews 1984: 31–2).[1] Yet in daily interactions and relationships with other children and with adults, children confront issues of justice, equal distribution and sharing. They respond to others' actions and feelings, and meet approval or disapproval of their own actions: 'morality is a fundamental, natural and important part of children's lives from the time of their first relationships' (Damon 1990: 1). Jerome Kagan (1986: xiii) argues that children are 'prepared' to make moral judgements (in the same sense that children are prepared – or 'programmed' – to speak) and that emotions are the basis for moral development. He quotes David Hume: 'Feelings, not reason, lie at the heart of morality.'

Not just parents, but also social scientists observe that children are sociable from the word go. In their early months they respond to and initiate interaction with parents and their elder sib, imitate her actions and interact playfully, angrily or aggressively with her (Dunn 1984: Ch. 2; Alderson 2000a: Ch. 2). These interactions form the basis for the beginnings of social understanding, of other people's intentions, feelings and needs. It is through experience that children learn to reason. Kagan suggests that children start to make moral judgements at about two years, that since at that age children also learn to talk, and talking requires prior maturation of cognitive abilities, it is likely that sensitivity to right and wrong cannot appear until children can infer possible states in others and also anticipate adults' reactions to their actions (Kagan 1986: x; Kagan and Lamb 1986). Damon adds that the development of children's natural engagement with moral issues (that is, through dealing with cases) benefits from adult guidance, and suggests that it may be in the fourth year that 'a combination of natural empathic awareness and reasoned adult encouragement leads the child to develop a firm sense of obligation to share with others' (1990: 35).

Matthews uses his philosophical discussions with children aged 8–11 (1980, 1984) to illustrate children's reasoning abilities and their enormous enthusiasm for such discussions, and his work has been an important part of an initiative (at the Institute for the Advancement of Philosophy for Children, in New Jersey) to introduce philosophy into schools (Pritchard 1996: Ch. 3). Matthews' approach to moral development (1987) has great advantages over the cognitive–developmental approaches of Piaget and Kohlberg (critiqued in Pritchard 1996: Ch. 8; Matthews 1994: Chs 4, 5). Thus Matthews argues that children are moral agents (rather than pre-moral persons), who develop a working knowledge of moral concepts at an early age – they do this through consideration of cases they encounter. As they get older – and encounter more cases and consider these – they enlarge and refine these concepts (rather than displacing them). Very importantly, Matthews sites children together with adults in a social world where they share encounters with moral issues, and thus he reduces the gap between adults and children.

Thomas Reid (an eighteenth-century Scottish philosopher) provides the starting point for Michael Pritchard's discussion of *Reasonable Children* (1996). Reid argued that the development of the powers of the mind, like bodily development, is 'the work of nature', but both benefit from encouragement and practice; and Pritchard argues that schools (as well as parents) can help children develop 'their powers of mind'. He develops a useful distinction between rationality and reasonableness, and also links between the two. The ability to think through an issue, and to provide reasons for one's beliefs and actions is part of both, but reasonableness has an extra dimension: it is primarily a social disposition. Pritchard quotes (with approval) this summary of the abilities and dispositions of a reasonable person:

> The reasonable person respects others and is prepared to take into account their views and their feelings, to the extent of changing her own mind about issues of significance, and consciously allowing her own perspective to be changed by others. She is, in other words, willing to be reasoned with.
> (Splitter and Sharp 1995: 6; quoted in Pritchard 1996: 3)

These abilities and dispositions may be developed and enlarged over time, but it is clear that young children possess them.[2] Judy Dunn's (1988) observational work shows how through experience of situations they face at home and through conversations with their mothers and sibs, young children engage with moral issues. As I shall show in this chapter, older children demonstrate in their accounts strong feelings of commitment to family members and responsibility for their welfare; their feelings lie at the heart of morality. The concept 'sentient activity' has been developed to harness together such feelings and actions that may arise from them (Mason 1996);

this concept builds on and moves on from the division of people work into 'caring about' (emotion) and 'caring for' (action) (Graham 1983). Sentient activity, as a composite concept, is especially useful for discussing children's moral engagement within family relations, since their strong feelings cannot always be matched with action. Their minority social status may inhibit action. But even a small action – comforting a tired mother – carries great emotional and moral weight, as mothers testify (see Mayall 1996: 69–74).[3]

Most of the work aimed at identifying children's moral knowledge and agency has used adult-controlled methods. Adults have asked young people to answer a questionnaire on moral issues (e.g. Shweder *et al.* 1986) or to discuss hypothetical situations, with adult prompts (e.g. Matthews 1984), or have observed and interpreted children's naturally occurring activities and interactions (e.g. Edwards 1986; Dunn 1988). Some recent work in the 'new childhood studies' has tried to reduce adult input into data-collection and to upgrade young people's input, by considering their own reflections on events in their own lives and on issues they identify in their own relationships. Here, initially, I aim to demonstrate moral agency through quoting a conversation. It is typical of young people's expressed moral competence, though, in response to dramatic events, gives a particularly detailed discussion.

Sandra, Karen and Anna

Sandra (aged 12) lived with her mother, brother (14) and new baby sister; Karen lived with her mother and four younger sibs. The two girls were friends and they chose to talk with me together. The example details dramatic events, which powerfully activated their thoughts. In discussing what emerges, I have concentrated mostly on Sandra. Just before this excerpt, the two girls talked about mothers' responsibility for childcare, and how their own health affects this. Karen's mother hurt her arm badly and has it in plaster, Sandra's mother recently had a Caesarean delivery and is depressed. Sandra says she doesn't like being a child, because there are conflicts between her child's right to go out to play, and her mother's need for help with the baby and housework. Then she tells the story of the birth and its implications for subsequent life at home.

> *Interviewer*: And your Mum, Sandra?
> *Sandra*: It was on the Thursday.
> *Interviewer*: Where were you?
> *Sandra*: My brother and me we had to go to the hospital with her. And I was going to come back to school on the Friday, because it was a Thursday, but I didn't because she had a Caesarean.

Interviewer: They didn't expect that?

Sandra: No, she had like pre-eclampsia and coliostasis and they had to start her off and they thought it might be stillborn, and it was like, she was in labour from like 12 till 10 at night and the baby nearly died – her heart-beat went right down, and they had to rush her in and take the baby out.

Interviewer: Were you there all this time?

Sandra: Yes, but we had to be most of the time in the waiting room. My Mum was getting really upset with all the time waiting for her.

Interviewer: And then what?

Sandra: Well, when she went in, we was like crying cos we thought the baby was dying. And my Mum was crying.

Interviewer: And did they look after you at all in the hospital?

Sandra: When my Mum was going in, she gave us £30 each, she felt sorry for us because we was having all this, and she gave us £30 [bit about central London hospital where the baby was born].

Karen: That's where my Mum was in. Cos my nextdoor neighbour called the ambulance and she got rushed up to the [local hospital] and they didn't have no stuff for the op, so that had to take her down to [central London hospital], and then they, she got picked up by an ambulance and taken down there. But she never had no painkillers nor nothing for it.

Sandra: And my Mum bought us all these crisps and magazines and stuff, but we didn't eat nothing.

Interviewer: Did the nurses look after you at all?

Sandra: They came and checked on us, but my Mum was having a really bad time and they had to stay with her most of the time. And there was loads of other people as well.

Interviewer: And once the baby had finally arrived?

Sandra: We was waiting in the waiting room and my Mum had the Caesarean about 15 minutes later, and the nurse came out with the baby and we held her, not even a minute old. And then we had to go home cos it was 12 o'clock at night and my Mum got my uncle to come and pick us up in his car.

Interviewer: Your Mum organized this after having the Caesarean? She made the phone call?

Sandra: No, she got the nurse to make the phone call. And I stayed at my friend's house for a couple of days and I didn't come to school on the Friday. And we come to the hospital every day, so. I was happy when the baby was first born –

Karen: And she's really cute –

Sandra: But now it's annoying, because she's always crying. It's like, we thought she was dying and she [the nurse] brought her and we –

Interviewer: She was ok.

Sandra: Yes, because my Mum only put a few stones on and they thought she was going to be really small, about four pounds, but she come out eight pounds four, and so –

Karen: That's a big baby.

Sandra: And we thought, but now when she cries my Mum has to do it all, because we don't like it any more. We're bored with her.

Interviewer: That's what you said at the outset, that as a mum you can't walk away from it. You've got to do it.

Sandra: Yes, when she's crying, my Mum's got to hold her and cook the dinner at the same time. And my Mum doesn't go out, she stays in all the time. The only time she goes out is when she goes shopping, or when she goes down the road to get a bottle of drink for her dinner.

Karen: And when my Mum wants to go shopping she has to take all the kids with her.

Interviewer: You don't stay at home by yourselves at all?

Karen: Not really. Sometimes me and my sister – yes, but not the little ones. Or if we stay at home, our nextdoor neighbour comes in and watches us.

Sandra: I sometimes look after my sister [the baby] for an hour like, if she has to go to the doctor. Cos she has to go regularly for check-ups. Cos she's got postnatal depression and she has to have regular check-ups for her scar. They say, Take three months off – blah, blah, but because she's got postnatal depression it'll take longer.

Interviewer: Is she really sad?

Sandra: She doesn't feel it all the time, but she says, when everything piles on top of her, with my brother watching TV all the time and the baby's crying and she's trying to get dinner, clean up, washing everything up, it's like, my Mum's a cleaning freak, so she likes to see everything done. And then she gets depressed then and she shouts at me for nothing sometimes. And I don't like it.

Interviewer: And can you help her in any way?

Sandra: Um, if we help out, like if the baby's crying, instead of saying, Mum, the baby's crying, just go and pick her up. Or if there's loads of dishes in the sink, don't say, Mum shall I wash the dishes, just go and wash a few dishes. Just to help her, cos there's lots of things get my Mum down, get on top of her . . . Sometimes I moan about it.

Sandra later explained that her mother's situation was especially hard because she had just been recovering from depression and thinking that she could go back to work as a nurse and that things would be financially better, when she 'fell pregnant'. And her mother's unhappiness was compounded because none of the fathers of the three children are on the scene or help out; the mother is angry when one of them occasionally turns up and gives a child 'a fiver and thinks that's going to be all right'.

Later on in the conversation I asked the girls how far they organized their use of time:

Sandra: Yes, I decide when I'm going out to play. And my Mum can't tell me where to go or who to play with. I decide by myself.

Interviewer: How long do you spend doing that?

Sandra: Well, if I have to help my Mum sometimes, I stay in after school for the whole time. But my Mum doesn't think it's fair on me to always have to help her, so she says I can go out if I want.

Here she demonstrates three parallel and intersecting strands in the child–adult relationship: her resentment against her mother's attempts to control her time out of the home, her participation in helping her mother – whether willingly or unwillingly, and her mother's recognition of a child's right to free time and time outside the home.

Sandra's account vividly demonstrates the processes whereby people's knowledge of the past shapes their moral responses in the present and on into the future. She has acted as her mother's confidante and knows about her mother's history, current circumstances and the progress of her feelings. This knowledge enables her to feel intense participant empathy for her mother's endurance and distress during the childbirth and in the months since then. Sandra also engages with ideologies of childhood – tensions between the normative and experiential. The mother provided for and protected her children through the childbirth process (giving money and arranging a lift home), but expects Sandra to participate in childcare and housework. Sandra understands how child–adult relations have changed since the baby's birth. The baby is a source of joy to the mother, but imposes stressful demands on both mother and daughter, who have to rethink their relations and contributions in the light of the baby's presence.

The story of these events shows clearly Sandra as a moral agent: she thinks through the complex implications of events for her behaviour; she knows that what she does makes a substantial difference to her relationship with her mother, to the management of the home and to her mother's ability to care for the baby. Sandra also demonstrates that she is coming to terms with a new relationship: having a new sister, someone whom she can look after and care about and for whom she can take some responsibility. She is also working through how best to live her days, in the light of family needs and normative ideas about childhood.

People's predispositions interlinked with past relationships also feed into the present interaction (cf. Bhaskar 1979: Ch. 3). It seemed that Karen had a happier outlook on life (she said childhood was 'great'); her relationship with her mother was perhaps easier, for she suggested that her mother was relatively happy and so needed less help from Karen; and she had a visiting stepdad whom she liked. Sandra had perhaps built up resentment against her mother; she had lived with her mother's depression before the pregnancy, through the pregnancy, childbirth and the baby's early months, and said her mother sometimes turned on Sandra and shouted at her 'for no reason'. Relations with fathers were also difficult; the mother was angry and resentful against the children's fathers' neglect, and she left it up to Sandra to contact her father – which she was unwilling to do. So some of Sandra's resentment focuses on her experience of intersections of gender and generation. Within the household, her brother failed to contribute to the family's well-being; she described him as lazy, unhelpful and selfish; he was also uninterested in schoolwork and wanted to leave school as soon as possible. Sandra, as I know from other evidence, was working as well as she could at school, and saw school education as important; she noted twice during the conversation that she had had to miss school during the childbirth episode, partly to show how serious the episode was, but partly also because she felt committed to school. Sandra's experience of family relationships has taught her a hard lesson: that mothers and daughters take responsibility for family welfare and for making what they can of opportunities.

Sandra's account contrasts with that given by Anna, a girl in the same class. She lived with her mother, stepfather and stepbrother (2.5 years), and went some weekends to stay with her father.

Anna: He comes to get me at the weekend. Sometimes I don't go, most of the times I do. He comes late on Friday, and I have my bath and go and go straight to bed when I get there.

Interviewer: Is it long since he moved?

Anna: Not really, about three years ago. And he asked me before if I wanted to live there, he asked me if I wanted to live in London and go there every weekend and I said, Yes. Cos he's got like two other children, they're my half-sisters. So I go there at weekends . . . So I get to see both parts of my family . . .

Interviewer: And what do you think it's like being a stepdad?

Anna: I think it must be quite good, because he treats me like his child and, like, I go to his family's house.

Interviewer: You've got three families!

Anna: Yes, and I love that, cos I get to have all different experiences . . . And he gives me my pocket money and buys me Christmas presents, and just, like, normally treats me like my own Dad does. He disciplines me. And if I'm scared or something. He helps me with my homework if I don't understand something. [Section here on how she plays out with her mates.]

Interviewer: So you have a lot of independence?

Anna: Yes. My Mum doesn't mind where I go provided I tell her where I'm going. So if my friends I'm hanging round with say, Let's go down to [x], I either phone my Mum or I go home and ask my Mum if I can go and have some money to go with. And if she says, No, that means no – I'm not going; then I stay in and watch TV or just go out to play in my area, but if she says, Yes, I do, I get what I need and go to [x].

Interviewer: Do you get money regularly so you can go by bus and –

Anna: Yes.

Interviewer: Is that irrespective of what you might have to do?

Anna: I do housework, I clean dishes, do the Hoovering. But sometimes I get money for it, it depends on, if I've been really good the whole week. But occasionally if I need money my Mum will give it me if she's got it. But if she's got like £1 in her purse she'll say, OK take it. But I'll say, No, it's OK I'll stay in . . .

Interviewer: So do you get on with your Mum – cos you said you did with your, both your fathers?

Anna: Yes, she's my best friend.

Interviewer: What sorts of things do you do with her?

Anna: I go out with her, to visit friends. I went with her to see the *Titanic*. And when my stepdad's out, we watch videos, we move the couch in front of the TV and we get loads of snacks and we watch TV, stuff like that, we watch movies together. [Section about gender issues at school.] I like school, I love coming to school. I don't want to leave school ever!

Interviewer: Are there some things you specially like about school?

Anna: I like being with my friends. I like most of my lessons, but there's no particular. I like dance and PE [more about subjects at school, and afterschool clubs, and a homework club].

Interviewer: So school's an important part of your life?

Anna: Yes. Most people just go home after school. They think I'm mad because I stay on. But sometimes I walk home with my friends, and then I get all my homework done and then I go out. And, like, every night I get my bag ready, so when I get up I can just [set off to school with it].

Interviewer: Yes, so is it up to you how you arrange your time after school?

Anna: Yes, so long as I let my Mum know.

Anna's account, of which these excerpts give only a taste, resonates with contentment about her family life, school life and life with her friends. She seems happy with her relationships with her three parents, enjoys what the home and school offers, and has enough free time away from home and school, with a good group of friends. It seems that her mother, father and stepfather have sorted out their own lives, or that they do not tell Anna their problems; they provide her with a reliable framework for her life, a framework which has been established and operationalized for several years.

Anna therefore is enabled by her circumstances to feel in charge of her life. The adults surrounding her facilitate her agency in family relationships. The negotiations she details about going out seem to take place on the basis of mutual trust – her mother is happy for her to go out with friends, but she in turn understands that on some occasions there is good reason for her to stay in. She can act responsibly towards getting an education, and plans to go to college later on.

We can see in these accounts relational processes whereby structures and agents interact. The established relationships, understandings and material conditions provide Sandra, Karen and Anna with a foundation on which to build their lives – taking account of their own history, predispositions, long-term goals, and immediate wishes. In working their way through current demands, current relationships, they in part reproduce, but in part transform the structures which mediate their thoughts and actions (cf. Archer 1998).[4]

Environments for moral agency

In this section I consider young people's moral agency in three main environments, the school, the neighbourhood and the home. Differing and distinctive processes in these environments shape their moral status – which they variously accept or contest.

School

As I discussed in Chapter 5, childhood in minority world countries may be described as scholarized, that is, children's 'proper' activity is as schoolchildren. I noted, too, that in England and Wales the separation of social elites from state education, and the ascription of responsibility for children's 'performance' at state schools to these non-élite mothers, have led to a climate of suspicion about the motivation and behaviour of children and their mothers, also of teachers and local education authorities. The low status of state school children – their minds and bodies – was indicated by the poor social and material conditions of their schools. Young people regarded schools as adult-led, and controlled by top-down education policies. These points indicate that the school environment is not conducive to respect for young people's moral agency.

Young people as pupils or as students?

The moral status of young people at school relates in important ways to their positioning as people in primary school or secondary school, in relation to teachers. In the Childhood Study, young people at North Secondary School reflected on changes in their experience at school now, compared to their primary school days.

In summary, at primary school, you have one teacher, you know her well and relate to her through your knowledge of her character – her virtues and failings, good and bad moods, personal circumstances – and in turn primary school teachers get to know the children and help them with their work. 'Pupils' find themselves morally subordinate to the teacher: following instructions and being helped, but the child–adult relationship is somewhat individual and personal.

At secondary school, you have many teachers and hardly know them as people at all; teachers expect the young people to behave as students – to listen, carry out tasks and take more responsibility for their own work; some teachers are unhelpful, unresponsive, others listen and respect students' views. 'Students' say they are asked to take more responsibility for their work, and so may think they have higher moral status, but their relations with teachers are more distant and formal. These are relations mainly between social positions – student as apprentice and teacher as authority; there is less opportunity for students to influence teacher–student interactions, since the relationship is not personal.

In group discussions at North Secondary School, where I suggested two topics, decision-making and taking responsibility, young people responded by discussing the home as the relevant site. When prompted to consider their agency at school, they generally emphasized that 'teachers have to make decisions for you' and 'you just do what you're told'. The few examples they gave of their own decision-making were not about central educational issues, but about what to play at break-times and what to eat at lunchtimes. Some identified small-scale examples of choice in lesson times – for instance, in PE 'you can pick your own team'. Later on, since students in earlier sessions had raised the issue of respect between children and adults, I prompted them to comment on respect at school.

Interviewer: At school do you get some kind of respect?
Steve: Sometimes we get respect, but not a lot of the time.
Bill: Other times –
Steve: We only get respect when they [the teachers] want to.
Bill: But if we don't respect them, they won't respect us.
Steve: Yes, but it's the same with the teachers; they've got to respect us. Say the teachers tell us to do all these things and then start shouting at us –
Harinder: Yes.
Bill: Yes.
Steve: They don't respect us.
Interviewer: No?
Steve: They don't respect anyone.
Harinder: They tell you to do a whole lot of things and they don't tell you exactly what to do and then –
Steve: Exactly. They give you instructions in Spanish or French or –
Harinder: And, I don't know, and they say, Just get on and work! [laughter]
Steve: And you put your hand up and they say, Put your hand down! And an hour later they come over and check it with you [laughter].

The excerpt shows their familiarity with the concept of mutual respect as a basis for relationships – which features prominently in the handbook issued to each student when they start at the school.

As in many of these discussion sessions, the young people delighted in developing a dramatic discourse, but they were indeed describing interactions which I observed during days with the class. The teacher would ask the class to carry out new and sometimes difficult tasks and then could not give help quickly to the many questioners. The students would talk with each other (about the work and about their own concerns) and teachers shouted above the noise – giving commands, reprimanding, marshalling.

In another group discussion, four students gave a succinct list of what makes a good teacher:

Interviewer: What is it about some of them that makes you get on better with them?
They just respect us and they give fun lessons.
And they don't have no favourites.
And they don't, like, pick on people and blame them . . .
Interviewer: How do they do it, the ones who do it well?
They listen to what you say.
And they don't rush you, and they tell you to take your time.
And they help you out, say if you get stuck . . .

Respect, fairness, understanding, listening and helpfulness were good teacher attributes, and taking the trouble to make lesson-times fun and well paced. Why teachers behave as they do is a large subject.[5] Here I just note current problems affecting their behaviour: demands made by the National Curriculum that teachers relay large amounts of information to young people who resist their lowly status, coupled with large classes in small spaces.

Schools as democratic institutions?
In the current educational climate, the prospects for democracy in schools in England and Wales look slight (Alexander 2000: Ch. 6). Young people are positioned essentially as the moral inferiors of teachers, the more competent in control of the less competent. In a large-scale survey of British schools, Priscilla Alderson (1999b) found that:

Pupils generally had low expectations of receiving fair treatment at school. Only a quarter said yes, they thought their teachers believe what they say, another half said this varies. About a third would trust a teacher to keep a secret and thought that teachers are careful to be fair before talking about pupils, and that they listen before deciding someone is at fault.

The survey revealed that half the students said they had a school council; 20 per cent thought it was effective and 28 per cent said it was ineffective. Virginia Morrow (2000) similarly reports on young people's verdicts on their school council; the selection of representatives from each year group was made by teachers rather than by the year group; suggestions and requests at the meetings were not taken up; the council was a token gesture rather than a force for improvement.

There has been a continuing tradition in the UK of argument in favour of democratizing schools (e.g. Meighan 1995; Meighan and Siraj-Blatchford 1997: Chapters 29–31; see also Apple and Beane 1999 for the USA).[6] And there are reported examples in Britain of schools which have democratized themselves (and probably many more go unreported). For instance, a head-teacher improved her school, which had had many behaviour problems, by facilitating the children's participation in working with staff to share agreements about rules and plans to improve the school; an Ofsted report enthusiastically noted that these work practices demonstrated the school's respect for the children and also served to improve behaviour (Highfield Junior School 1997).

Two teachers at an infant school give an inspiring account of how they worked in participation with children on the inside and outside spaces. They explain:

> It has been our intention to give the young children in our care some personal responsibilities and some choice. The children learn to respect the few rules we impose and see the sense of them, and we notice how they care for and watch out for one another when they are outside . . . We believe that children at work and play in a lively, changing and diverse landscape will react imaginatively and build up high expectations and happy recollections of school life.
>
> (Humphries and Rowe 1994: 116)

At a secondary school, Carter (2000) found through discussions with boys that they lacked self-esteem; through group work he helped them to value themselves and what they could do, and enabled them to feel they had contributions to make to class discussions. Somewhat similarly, Cunningham (2000) learned from students that they did not feel able to contribute to class discussions unless they felt safe from ridicule from other students; collaborative work between students and teachers began to establish an ethos of respect within classrooms, so that all might contribute actively in exchanging views. But Cunningham notes that students rarely tried to discuss the curriculum itself; students these days tend to think there is no mileage for change there.

But another study points to recent anti-democratic trends in education. This followed a cohort of children who started primary school in 1991 through to the top year (Triggs and Pollard 1998). This cohort was the first to be exposed to the full vigour of governmental changes – the National Curriculum, national testing at 7 and 10, competition between schools. As the years passed, fewer children valued being able to choose – that is, be active learners – and fewer enjoyed the core curriculum. Increasingly as they got older, the children explained that the teacher knew what they had to learn, that their futures depended on them learning these things, and that exploratory, active, participative work by them would waste valuable time (Triggs and Pollard 1998: 112–18). The general message is that in the present climate of top-down, highly controlled instruction, children are losing confidence in their own learning.

Many UK studies find that schools are profoundly undemocratic, and that young people experience rejection of their moral agency. Yet if moral competence is acquired through interactive experience and if adults have a part to play in guiding young people, then teachers, surely, should engage with young people in discussing moral issues. It will be counter-productive simply to tell them how democracy works, for then they will see ever more clearly how undemocratic their school is. Young people's engagement with moral issues must include studying the school as an institution, and in planning and managing democratic improvements to it (Pritchard 1996; Alderson 1999a; Osler 2000).

Neighbourhood and public spaces

Researchers have tackled young people's experiences of their neighbourhoods and use of public space, and are confirming what common experience suggests: that the mutually reinforcing processes of protection and exclusion are altering the experiences of young people. They feel that they are not accepted as rightful users of public space, that adults think they are in the wrong place at the wrong time, and that adults suspect their motives.

Margaret O'Brien (2000) reports on young people's use of public space in inner London, outer London and new town areas, using a large-scale questionnaire and neighbourhood case studies. The young people were aged 10/11 and 13/14. There was wide variation in use of public space, though those living in the new town had more access than Londoners. Gender and ethnicity were relevant: older girls of Asian background were most likely to be restricted.[7] As compared to data from 1970, there was a dramatic decline in 10/11-year-olds going to school unaccompanied by an adult (from 94 to 47 per cent).

Gill Valentine (1999) found that parents (of 8–11-year-olds) worry about traffic and strangers. They take account of their child's perceived competence rather than age when assessing whether to let their children out. Children's access to public space has to be constantly negotiated, and they sometimes find ways of bypassing parental consent.

Virginia Morrow (2000) found in group discussions with young people (12–15 years) about their neighbourhoods that they identified some good places, but rather more bad features of their environments: racism, dirty open spaces, traffic-ridden streets. Thus not having a safe, decent place to play was one important theme. A second theme was that they 'felt mistrusted and not respected by the adults around them' (Morrow 2000: 146), both at school and in their neighbourhoods. Third, they felt excluded from decision-making at community level. Morrow notes that this is a bleak picture of non-participation and poverty of environment for the young people, but that family and friends were positive sources of support, trust and company.

Hugh Matthews and colleagues (2000) found that young people (mainly aged 12–16) interviewed in shopping malls in midlands English towns tended to come there regularly. These were warm, bright places, with a certain 'buzz', for teenagers to 'hang out' in. In particular, they were safe places for girls, but 70 per cent of the young people thought they were under adult surveillance and 44 per cent had the experience of 'being moved on', with more boys than girls (57 versus 39 per cent) suffering this. Whilst it seemed that adults regarded young people's group presence in public space as suspicious, they themselves resisted their exclusion from it, and assumed 'the mantle of the hybrid':

> Here young people are no longer child [sic], living within the safe haven of the home, nor quite adult, with powers to move freely and unassailably within the public domain. By locating themselves in settings that transgress and so question the spatial hegemony of adult-hood, young people journey into the interstitial territory of thirdspace.
>
> (Matthews *et al.* 2000: 292)

Young people's dubious status in public space extends to how they are treated in shops; a study found that they were commonly pushed aside by adults, who assumed they should be served first. Young people (aged 11 and 12) argued strongly that the principle of fairness should apply equally to them as to adults (Brannen *et al.* 2000: 29–33).

These studies resonate with my data from the 1990s. As noted in Chapter 4 (p. 55), traffic danger and stranger danger were fundamental concerns for parents, against which they weighed their children's competence and 'read-iness' to use public space. In the Childhood Study, where 9-year-olds reported on their use of public space unaccompanied by an adult, gender issues emerge clearly. Girls were more restricted, whatever their ethnicity.

If you put together the two classes (at East and North Schools), more boys than girls went out to play, or to the shops or park, and more went

Table 6.1 Children out unaccompanied by adult (East and North Primary Schools 9-year-olds, Childhood Study)

	Out to play		To school		
	Yes	*No*	*No*	*Yes*	*Number*
Girls	11	14	17	8	25
Boys	25	7	12	20	32
All	36	21	29	28	57

to school not accompanied by an adult, but alone or with friends or sibs (see Table 6.1).

However, moving on to secondary school was a break point; young people themselves wished to travel there unaccompanied, and most parents in both the Risk and Childhood Studies allowed it. The social unacceptability of being accompanied to secondary school is linked up in the minds of parents and young people with changes in social status of people called 'teenagers', who are the majority of secondary school attenders (for my respondents in the Childhood Study, 'teenager' means 13 years and upwards). As two 12-year-old girls note, in their discussion of the social status of 'teenager':

Sally: They've got more choice really. They're old enough to take decisions. Your parents think you are old enough to make decisions. And by now, they still take care of you, but they think you can take care of some things yourself.

Rebecca: You're more responsible. And they're still overprotective. At any age they are, my Mum says. They think the worst if you're not there or –

Interviewer: You say overprotective – do you think too protective?

Sally: We say overprotective, but our parents are only doing it for our good.

(North Secondary School, Year 8)

Notably however, girls of Asian descent (aged both 9 and 12) were mostly accompanied to and from school. These girls spent their time out of school with family – at home and at relative's homes. Most of the other 12-year-olds were allowed out. But whilst most of the girls reported that they had to negotiate for permission each time (as Sandra and Anna indicated earlier in this chapter), boys were much freer to choose for themselves.

These studies have some common themes. First, in adults' discourse and behaviour, children are understood as potential victims, of traffic and strangers, but also as potential threats, as people in the wrong place; they do not have legitimacy, they may be up to no good. Recent legislation has set in place curfews for under-10s; however no local authority has implemented these (Gill 2001).[8]

Second, in our society, it seems we regard adults as responsible for children in public places; children are either not present on their own account or are there under licence from parents. The exclusion of children from public space has been noted as a growing trend in western societies (Ward 1978, 1988; Zelizer 1985; Cahill 1990; Hillman 1993; Engelbert 1994).

Third, gender matters in young people's usage of public space. It is clear that restrictions on use of outside space are more complete for girls than for boys, and especially for girls of Asian origin. Though Matthews and colleagues (2000) argue that adults understand public space as freely available for adults, there is competing evidence that many women understand public space as hostile to women; it belongs to men rather than to all adults (Little *et al.* 1988).

Home

Young people's access to public space leads on to considering how people judge the quality of their home lives. At issue here is how people value independence and interdependence.

The fact that young people argue for freedom to go out is an expressed need for activity, with friends usually, beyond the home; this can be interpreted as a wish for independence. But many young people (aged 9/10 and 12/13, Childhood Study) valued interdependence, solidarity with the family – 'being with my family' and 'family times'. They enjoyed the experience and cementing of family relations.[9] Close identification with the family – its history, culture, its future, relationships, means that these London young people felt part of it, and that implied contributing to helping it function, by participating in building and maintaining relationships, helping parents, doing chores, helping with younger sibs. It is through this emotional identification that moral agency develops.

Obedience and family work

As described in Chapter 4, most children first learn about their status as children through inhabiting the family, where people belong to two social groups: parents and children; children recognized and accepted parental authority and the child duty of obedience. Childhood Study conversations point to dependency and interdependence in relation to parents. At home, moral issues are central to children's experience, learning and activity. Here, for instance, are two 9-year-olds talking, in reply to opening gambits about what it is like being a child:

> *Grace*:   You have to obey, up to grown ups . . .
> *Janice*:   You can't do whatever you want to do, until you're 18 or 16. You have to ask permission, and you haven't got so much money. You only get pocket money and that's for school.
> *Grace*:   And you have to go home early after school, or if you're playing outside you have to get in at a certain time.
> *Interviewer*: And in your case, what time is that?
> *Grace*:   I don't know. It depends when my Mum calls me.
> *Interviewer*: And are there some times when you think of yourselves as children?

Janice:	Yes, I do. Because if I wasn't a child, I'd be doing some stuff of my own. I wouldn't be having to go asking my Mum all the time. I could do what I wanted . . .
Interviewer:	And are there times when you think you're not a child?
Janice:	I am a child, but when I have to look after my sister [aged 2], my Mum goes, You're a big girl now, you must look after your sister. But sometimes she goes, You're too small to go there. And I don't understand. Sometimes she says, You're a big girl and sometimes she says, You're a small girl – you can't do that.
Grace:	My Mum, my Dad, sometimes my Mum says the same to me. When it comes to tidying up, she says, You're a big girl, you should tidy up, but when it comes to playing outside she says, You're small.

(North Secondary School, Year 8)

It is through obedience, in this conversation, that the girls learn to contribute to the family work order, doing childcare and housework. Almost all the 9-year-olds did some chores and many describe this as a means of 'giving Mum a break'. The North 9-year-olds did chores and childcare, some routinely and others on occasion. North 12-year-olds mostly took delegated, routine responsibility for jobs. There was a somewhat different pattern in the East schools, where part of socialization into family culture is learning to do the jobs, especially for girls. In many of these families, with parents working very long hours, including mothers doing machining work at home, children's contributions were even more essential.

Children as confidants

Though moral actions may result from obedience, it became clear that young people often initiate good deeds. Many young people acted as confidants, notably to mothers. For instance, Janet (age 9) lives with her mother and baby sister in a cramped flat. She shares the only bedroom with her sister. Her mother sleeps in the sitting room. Janet says she doesn't get enough space and time, because her mother wants time to herself and so asks Janet to look after the baby. Janet knows a lot about her mother's history (two non-resident fathers, poverty, unhappiness), acts as confidante and somewhat on equal terms as friend to her mother.

Janet:	Well, sometimes, I think it's OK cos I like my sister, but sometimes I want my own space, cos she's always taking it off all the time . . . And my Mum is always too busy, and, like, when she [Mum] has got time of *her* own, I have to do something – and when I'm looking after my sister,

my sister's always with me. And I want my own space.
Cos with my own friends, I have to play with them while
she's got the Teletubbies on.

Interviewer: And does your time include doing jobs around the place?

Janet: Yes, I make my Mum a cup of tea, be her servant – let her
borrow my money [laughs].

Interviewer: You get on well with her?

Janet: Yes, but she is annoying. Cos she borrows my money on
a Saturday and says she'll pay it back on Thursday . . .

Interviewer: And you're company for her?

Janet: Yes, cos she tells me all her problems. And if she's watching a film I sit with her until it's my bedtime, and when I
go, Ooh! sometimes I stay up late.

Interviewer: And so does she also need time on her own?

Janet: Yes, cos I wind her up and she winds me up and then,
and then my sister does. And sometimes I feel really angry
and I want to tell her.

Interviewer: You get angry with her?

Janet: Yes.

(North Primary School, Year 5)

Looking after Mum

Young people also responded to their identification of their mother's
needs for care. Caring includes caring about their mothers, but also more
practically providing care. Distressed mothers and ill mothers need looking after. A 'working' mother needs a cup of tea on her return home,
and help with the dishes. These 12-year-old boys' fathers had both
moved out; Leo lived with his brother, mother and stepfather; Rob with
his mother. (Girls talked like these boys too, but I quote boys here
because boys are often stereotyped as not emotionally involved and as
unhelpful.)

Interviewer: This bit about what sorts of things children are meant to
do [i.e. in the topic list]. You said go to school and do
homework, Leo. Anything else?

Leo: Chores.

Rob: Look after their mum.

Interviewer: What kinds of things do you do for her?

Rob: I do the washing up sometimes. When she wants me to
cook the dinner, I try to cook the dinner.

Leo: Try! [Laughter.]

Rob: And if she's not well, call the doctor.

Interviewer: And is she sometimes not well?

Rob: Well, like in January she had this dizziness thing, and when she woke up she felt so dizzy she couldn't stand up. So I called the hospital and they came and –

Interviewer: You called the hospital direct?

Rob: Yes.

(North Secondary School, Year 8)

Later Leo said he went after school to her place of work and they came home together. 'And then we come straight home and I make sure she's OK and make her tea and stuff.' And: 'Every day I do washing up, and tidying the house and Hoovering and stuff.' These boys, like others, emphasized their pleasure in family life: 'family times', shopping, expeditions.

Interviewer: What do you enjoy most about your life?

Rob: Christmas and birthday!

Leo: I like quite sentimental things, like when we go out for the day and do something together. Like on the weekend we went to Southend and had a game of crazy golf and that was really really nice. I quite like sentimental things, not just getting presents and stuff [joint laughter]. Cos the best thing I've had in my life is this [a St. Christopher's medal on a chain], cos my [step]dad gave it me and my brother's got one too. So, and when he gets things like combat gear and stuff, my Mum gets us it too, and sometimes we all go out with Arsenal T-shirts and combat. And she makes jokes about, look at my three boys and stuff.

Reciprocal relations

Young people commonly presented caring for parents as a component of reciprocal relations; they care for you, you care for them. Life-long responsibility for reciprocal caring was not overt in most young people's discourse, but it was an expressed and practised norm among those whose parents had, as the accounts showed, immigrated from societies where such interdependence is traditional. Ferdous is the eldest boy in a Muslim family where the parents came from Bangladesh; neither parent is in paid work. Mark lives with his mother, father and two younger brothers. Both are aged 12.

Interviewer: What are the good things about young people being with their parents?

Mark: It's fine. Your parents give you things. They help you in some ways, like if you don't understand something.

Interviewer: Do you do things for them?

Mark:	I – I look after my brother. What do you mean?
Interviewer:	Well, some people say they might make a cup of tea for their mum if she's tired.
Ferdous:	Well, I look after my father, because they can't speak very good English. So sometimes he needs help if he goes somewhere.
Interviewer:	So you act as interpreter?
Ferdous:	Yes.
Interviewer:	Are there any bad things about being in a family?
Mark:	No.
Ferdous:	No.
Mark:	If you didn't have a family, you couldn't have any fun like you can with your parents.
Ferdous:	And your mum and dad look out for you.
Mark:	They look after you. Because they don't want anything to happen to you.
Ferdous:	I don't want to leave my parents because they've been like sticking up for me and looking after me, and I want to give that back, because they're getting old and they'll need help. So I help them.

(North Secondary School, Year 8)

Working on the project of their own life

Young people's moral agency was also shown in their accounts of how they worked on the project of their own life, through relational processes. They described childhood as time when they fitted into the week: friendships and play, personal interests, social times at home, keeping up relationships with non-resident relatives, as well as doing schoolwork and jobs at home. An important process in the lives of these young people is negotiating the change from primary to secondary and the associated change to the new social status: teenager; these processes affect family relationships. Here are two 12-year-old boys discussing how they sometimes refuse to do chores and 'give their mum lip'.

Suraj:	Lately she [Mum] might say, I'm going to have to deal with these teenage symptoms coming up, cos I'm growing up and getting ratty, cos I'm getting thirteenager [*sic*].
Interviewer:	Do you think of yourself as someone who's becoming a teenager?
Suraj:	No! We just think of ourselves as Us!
Interviewer:	But your mothers think you are?
Peter:	Yes, cos my Mum thinks I'm getting all these symptoms, because these days I'm getting like lippy . . .

Interviewer: And do you get treated as children sometimes?
Suraj: Yes and no.
Interviewer: When are you?
Suraj: When you're told to do the dishes. She says, you should do the dishes cos you're young – it means you'll grow up to be a better person [laughing]. She says children are meant to do dishes. That's how she takes on . . .

(North Secondary School, Year 8)

Coping with change

Young people's accounts also indicate their moral agency in coping with major change in the family – which is commonplace in family life. For instance, of 29 young people in the North Primary Class, at least 12 had experienced or were currently living through major changes. These included: father leaving home; family moving house across country so the child lost friends; new stepfather and half-sibs moving in; mother's serial boyfriends; illnesses and deaths of grandparents; death of mother; parents working extra-long hours because of financial crises. Other major events included prolonged bullying at school, hospitalization for asthma, learning about mother's previous miscarriages and stillborn babies. Significantly, in line with the low moral status they understand as theirs, young people do not give themselves credit for this agency. But how do they cope with such events? Their accounts indicate a number of strategies. They discussed and worked through issues with their parents, especially mothers. They also talked with each other – as some of the excerpts given in this book show – and these conversations probably helped acceptance and coping. Being in a class where many others have faced change, and where there was a lot of discussion – encouraged by the teacher in class and carried on between themselves at break-times – was important. A critical ingredient was respectful child–adult relations and respectful relations between parents (compare Smart and Neale 2000a, 2000b).

General points

Some general points emerge from what the young people say. Their accounts all show how attached these 9- and 12-year-olds are to their family. This may seem obvious but it is important to note how their moral agency builds on their strong feelings (as discussed at the start of this chapter).

Second, it is clear that they understand the home as the social environment which is meant to create the moral person. Young people think moral training is a central parental function. The extent to which they can and do negotiate details varies according to parental notions of parent child relations – along a continuum from authoritarian to democratic.

Third, opportunities for moral agency are greater at home than at school. At school, young people refer to the relatively fixed structures; they may struggle as agents with these structures, but can make little change. The home, however, is the site of relational processes between the generations whereby children and parents make and remake the structures, that is, the relationships, family customs and activities, mutual understandings.

Recognizing and then respecting children's moral reasoning and agency is the gateway to respecting their participation rights. For children's rights to provision and protection are far more commonly respected than their participation rights, since by long tradition they are regarded as irrational and therefore incompetent (Alderson 1993: 32–5).

Accounting for the complexities of children's moral status

In this chapter, I have discussed young people's moral agency in child–adult relations. Gareth Matthews' account of how children from their early years build up and expand their moral knowledge over time, using cases, fits well with how the young people in my own and others' studies talked. Using examples, they demonstrated sophisticated understanding of childhood's moral status, and of how, in relation to that, they understood their own experiences and actions. They showed that they were reasonable people: they were both able and willing to take account of other people's views, they were willing to change their own views or actions responsively, and they could and did put aside their own immediate interests with the aim of helping others. Not surprisingly, they often did not give themselves credit for their own moral agency; in this they reflect children's low moral status in our society.

Thus they indicated there is a fault line between their moral competence in practice, and their ascribed low moral status – especially outside the home. Like women tackling the feminine mystique (see Smith 1988: Ch. 2), young people tried to come to terms with the 'childhood mystique' which invaded their consciousness; sometimes they downgraded their own moral status, at other times they fiercely resisted and asserted their competence. It is notable that their moral agency is clearly seen in their interactions with their mothers; women and children find common cause in difficult and oppressive social circumstances. Chapter 7 takes up the fault line theme, in discussing a child standpoint.

This chapter argues and demonstrates that the home is the main site where children's moral agency is both expected and enacted, whereas in school and in public places their moral status is low. In Chapter 7, I shall discuss moral agency in children's friendships. As Hutchby and Moran-Ellis (1998) argue children's moral competency is principally enacted in two contexts: at home and with friends. These are both out of the public gaze and difficult to study. One reason why children's moral status is low is that their agency is not visible to people whose opinions shape ideologies of childhood. The adults who know most about children's moral agency – mothers – are weakly positioned to speak for children. The power lies with psychological formulae, as outlined early in this chapter, and with influential professionals – doctors, social workers, health visitors, teachers, the legal professions – who rely on psychological descriptions as a basis for their work on, for and with children. [10]

And we also have to note that the long process over more than one hundred years, whereby young people have been removed from the labour force and sited as school pupils, has had a profound effect on adult understandings of childhood (Zelizer 1985). In Chapter 8, I compare some UK childhoods with some in Finland, where a number of other factors affect how childhood is understood; important among these is the idea that children contribute to the economy. In the UK, both the scholarization of childhood and its privatization – with children as dependants, hidden in the family – encourage the view that they do not engage in socially useful activities, and hence their moral agency is downgraded (cf. La Fontaine 1999).

There is, however, modest encouragement to be derived from the increasing number of studies that are examining children's agency, and that may in time help to shift ideas. In particular I am cheered by studies which are taking seriously young people's understandings of the 'teenage years', and showing that rather than seeking lonely autonomy, people value interdependence and allegiance to family beyond childhood. This helps us think of people relationally and as contributors, rather than as individual dependants. Studies in other cultures have earlier revealed interdependence as a key virtue, and research in the UK is now able to draw on the understandings of people whose roots lie in other cultures but who are making their way here (see also Ch. 4: 49).

7 | Towards a child standpoint

Introduction

Thus far, I have considered child–adult relations in the light of the generationing processes through which those defined as children and as adults interact. This chapter considers young people's understandings of childhood itself, still within its generational relations, but with emphasis on the constituent characteristics of childhood, on children as a social group, on how they deal with the social status of childhood. I take the stance, not of 'looking down', but of 'looking up'. This chapter moves towards consideration of the idea of a child standpoint (Hartsock 1983; Smith 1988, 1999; Harding 1991: 119–37). Feminist work is about another subordinated group – women, but the approach – giving due attention to people's experiences as a basis for analysing their social condition – is relevant to thinking about children. Young people's accounts of their experiences in their designated status as children, their evaluations of these, how far they perceive disjunctions between models of childhood they have learned and experience – these are the basis for analysis in this approach. Through this analysis one may move outwards from the local to identify those structures that shape their lives and explain processes: how and why it is that childhood is as it is, and is developing in certain ways.[1]

In this chapter, first I consider how young people describe the social status of childhood. Second, I discuss the idea of children as a minority social group. I then take the specific case of play as a feature of childhood. Finally, I discuss how we can move towards developing a child standpoint.

Childhood as social status

In the Childhood Study, I elicited young people's accounts, through discussion with them in pairs, about the social status of motherhood, fatherhood and then childhood. I asked them what it was like being (called) a child, what were the good and bad things about childhood; and whether their parents had expectations of them, and they of their parents (East and North 9-year-olds and North 12-year-olds).

There are inherent dangers in this approach. As Connell (1987: 54–66) has noted in the case of gender, to start off from categorizing people or experience as gendered is to make assumptions and to reify rather than to explore. More useful, he argues, is to consider processes whereby gendering is accomplished. In the case of generational relations, my earlier studies showed that young people do draw clear distinctions between childhood and adulthood, and that it was important to explore these distinctions with them. But during these research conversations, as I shall show, young people moved back and forth between the normative and processes in their experiences, justifying their normative points and checking and modifying them against experience. And later in the research process I also specifically asked them to consider relationships between their understanding of their social status and how things worked out in their daily lives.

Childhood as social status

> *Interviewer*: This bit here [in the topic list] about being a child? I'm not assuming you're a child.
> *Angela*: I *am* a child!
> *Joanne*: I think I'm a child.
> *Angela*: Because we don't really have any responsibilities do we?
> *Interviewer*: I don't know.
> *Angela*: Not like mums and dads. And we're not older, like 16 or 18, so we are children really.
> *Joanne*: We are children. Because children are the lowest. Like, there's adults and children but the adults are over you, on top.
>
> (North Secondary School, Year 8)

These girls outlined some of the main points made by both 9- and 12-year-olds: clear distinctions between childhood and adulthood as to responsibility, age, and hierarchy. Other points on childhood as social status made in these interviews include: restrictions, absence of rights, childhood as a time for learning, and protection and provision.

Donny: It's someone to love you and look after you, so you don't have to worry about anything, cos they do everything for you.

(North Secondary School, Year 8)

Josh: You don't have to work, you don't have to get money to live.
Peter: You don't have to buy your clothes and shoes.
Interviewer: You don't have to work?
Josh: Well, you see, like, your dad and mum are the people who go to work, and you just go to school to learn and you don't exactly have to, like when you're an adult you have to do much harder work.

(North Primary School, Year 5)

Hari: I think I'm mainly a child. You're only properly grown up when you're 18.
Interviewer: Why do you say that?
Hari: Cos that's when you're allowed to drink and buy a house and all that stuff.

(North Secondary School, Year 8)

Young people understood childhood comparatively – with adulthood. They drew on their experience in their own and other families to make general points. Through these conversations runs a pervasive view that childhood is relatively easy compared to adulthood, although adult control can be irksome.

Pros and cons of childhood

Privilege?

Interviewer: What's it like being a child?
Sabah: It's fun. If you're old, you can't do that much stuff, like riding bikes and exercises.
Shama: It's fun, because you play lots of games and when you're older you don't get that much time to play. And you have to do homework when you're in secondary school.
Interviewer: Do you have time to play?
Shama: Yes, when I've done my homework. [She explains her routine: home from school at 3.30, one hour to eat, mosque from 5 to 7, homework, then play, then dinner and bed at 10.]
Interviewer: And are there any bad things about being a child?

Sabah:	You get told off a lot.
Shama:	And you get on your mother's nerves when you do something wrong.

(East Primary School, Year 5)

The two girls identified an intrinsic and socially accepted activity of childhood: play. But the play activities of childhood were allowed for more in the primary school years than at secondary school. Being told off by mothers was the downside of childhood, but later on they spontaneously and enthusiastically described their close confiding relations with their mothers.

Interviewer:	I'm trying to find out what it's like being a child, except maybe you don't think of yourself as a child – maybe a person, or a boy?
Ravinder:	I'm a child!
Interviewer:	Why is that?
Ravinder:	Like, not a person, I'm a child of my Mum and Dad.
Interviewer:	And what about you?
Atiq:	Same.
Interviewer:	And are there good things about being a child?
Atiq:	You have fun at school.
Interviewer:	What sort of fun?
Ravinder:	Doing work like geography and art and painting and technology and doing the computer and playing.
Interviewer:	And are there any bad things about it?
Ravinder:	Yes, some. Like English – you have to write stories. It's a bit boring. He [teacher] gives you titles, he gives you four to choose from every week . . .
Interviewer:	And life at home – are there some good things?
Atiq:	Some, like playing with your friends in the street, and helping your mum and dad. One thing I don't like is when there's nothing to do.
Interviewer:	Are you more often bored at home than at school?
Atiq:	Yes. If I'm bored I just watch TV or walk about.
Ravinder:	If I'm good, I go outside and play, or read in my bedroom.

(East Primary School, Year 5)

Here, the first boy drew attention to the permanence of the child–parent relation. (Several of the 12-year-olds also noted that they were still treated as their parents' child, even though in other contexts, they regarded themselves as not children.) The boys focus on school as a fun time – though not in all subjects; and school provided interesting activities, whereas at home sometimes there was nothing to do. Some young people, discussing the same initial question, chose to focus on subordinate status:

Interviewer: What's it like being a child?

Sajid: You have to be good. You come to school every day. Respect the teacher.

Interviewer: Who says you have to be good?

Sajid: Teacher. And mums and dads.

Interviewer: Do they say that? 'Be good!'?

Sajid: Yes.

Interviewer: Are there good things about being a child?

Sajid: [Pause]

Interviewer: Are there bad things?

Sajid: Yes. You don't get spending money. Only at Diwali, you get about £100. My Mum gets it from her sisters, they give it her, right, like £10 and £5, and my Mum's got about £100 and then she gives me it.

Interviewer: So it's a good time of year?

Sajid: Yes.

Interviewer: So are there any bad things about being you?

Sajid: Not allowed to play out. Only sometimes. Saturday and Sundays.

Interviewer: Are you too busy during weekdays?

Sajid: Yes. I do my homework and then I go mosque and come back at 7 and do my homework.

Interviewer: Would you like things to be different?

Sajid: We don't get that much play-time.

(East Primary School, Year 5)

Sajid was leading a very strictly organized 'hard' life (see also Chapter 4 for the hard lives of Muslim boys). In respect of 'hardness' childhood was like adulthood, but key to child status were obedience and respect towards adults, and financial dependence. Childhood should include play-time, but his childhood did not allow enough of it.

The character of the talk at North Primary School was somewhat different. The young people also identified obedience as a feature of childhood, but discussed negotiation with parents to alter established daily routines.

Interviewer: What's it like being a child?

Ann: It's all right. It's quite good. You go to school and learn lots of things, more than your mum and dad, cos when they have children they can't really go to college cos they have to look after the children.

Gill: One of the bad things, cos when you want to see something [e.g. on TV], or do something like adults do, you get really jealous and then when you ask them they get angry and you can't do anything and you feel helpless.

Interviewer: Can you give some examples?

Gill: Like if your friends they walk home [unaccompanied by an adult] and you say, 'Can I do that?' and she says 'No'. And you feel really sad, cos you really want to do that.

Interviewer: Do you feel you have to do what you're told?

Ann: Well, you have to be really nice to them, and go, please, pleease!

Gill: And then they might let you. You have to do what you're told mostly.

Interviewer: Is this your mothers you're talking about, or is it all adults?

Ann: All adults. You have to do it. cos if you're disobedient you just get in more trouble. Like with X [their class teacher].

Interviewer: You do feel that, if she says so you have to?

Ann: Yes, if she says something then we have to do it.

(North Primary School, Year 5)

Ann started off with childhood as a time of opportunity, denied later in life, to go to school and learn things, but Gill, looking down the topic list to where I had listed the question: 'Are there any bad things about being a child?', immediately chipped in with her current problem – that her mother would not let her walk to school with friends. The personal issue was taken up in general terms by Ann, who noted that you have to adopt wheedling tactics to get a reasonable deal; Gill took this up and expanded the discussion to the general topic – obedience – which again Ann ran with – children have to obey not just mothers but adults in general.

This excerpt exemplifies how young people linked together the personal and the general. They defined a personal problem within wider child–adult relations. This next snippet shows how the direction of the conversation can go the other way – from the general to the particular. Bill was very talkative, and dominated the conversation; he was facing difficult times at home and used the research conversation to expound these.

Andrew: There are good things about being a mother, cos you've got children.

Bill: And my Mum can't cope without children. She says that. Because she's alone sometimes, and she needs children. And we always say, 'Mum, we'll look after you.' And she goes, 'I love you,' you know and all the rest.

(North Primary School, Year 5)

Bill was in a very small minority among my informants, since he could not always count on his mother's love, and he had experienced the frailty of adult relations – he had seen his mother dealing with rejection and neglect. He felt a serious responsibility for ensuring that his mother was surrounded by his care, whereas for most young people in this study, though they talked about caring for parents, the primary responsibility went the other way, from parent to child.

Dependence, lack of decision-making

Jane:	It's like, you can't wait till you're an adult, so you can do what you want.
Interviewer:	Cos you can't do what you want?
Jane:	No, you've got to ask your Mum.

(North Primary School, Year 5)

Interviewer:	And are there any bad times?
Lindsay:	Yes, when I can't get what I want.
Sarah:	Yes, cos if my Mum wants to go out and I want to stay in, and we end up going out. I have to do what I'm told.
Lindsay:	There's a few hard times. Cos if . . . you go out and play with your friends and you forget [the time] and then you go back [home] and your parents are angry.

(North Primary School, Year 5)

Interviewer:	Are there things you look forward to?
Chris:	Yes. Being 11, in two years, because I'll be older and then I'll get even older and then I can make my own decisions. That's why I want to be older.
Interviewer:	What would you like to make decisions about?
Chris:	About going out, whenever I want. When I'm 17, I'll be able to stay out late, not too late. I'll have to come back around 9, 10. When I'm older, not now.

(North Primary School, Year 5)

One of the main downsides of childhood was constantly having to ask permission, especially about going out.

Childhood as fun

Amy:	Yes, cos you can go to clubs, like in the school, and adults can't do that.
Trish:	Being a child for me is quite good because, I can't really explain it, but –
Amy:	You just enjoy it.
Trish:	Yes, you just enjoy it. And you get all subjects in school that you won't get when you grow up, like art.

(North Primary School, Year 5)

'You just enjoy it' – this was a common refrain. Further, children were capable of fun, whereas adults were less good at it. Normatively, childhood should have fun elements. More detail is added by these cheerful Year 8 boys.

Interviewer:	What do you value about your life at present?
Suraj:	It's freedom, innit? You don't have to worry about anything.
Steve:	Yes.
Interviewer:	No worries?
Suraj:	Yes, it's just happy. No strain, just getting up and learning.
Interviewer:	Do you like learning?
Suraj and Steve:	Yes.
Interviewer:	Do you like coming here and doing all this stuff?
Steve:	Yes, but I don't like getting up in the morning.
Suraj:	Getting up.
Interviewer:	But once you get here?
Steve:	Then it's OK cos all your friends are here.
Suraj:	And it feels better when you know more as well. You can go home and tell your parents about what you learned.

(North Secondary School, Year 8)

Life for them, currently, was free, happy, with no strain; learning was enjoyable and school provided days with your friends. These boys held to their theme even though I (being worried about adverse effects of current education policies on children's well-being) suggested my doubts to them. The corrective to my view was common:

> *Joe*: I like having an education and having my friends at school. I like coming to school. If you were at home, you can't hardly enjoy yourself like you can here.

(North Secondary School, Year 8)

But while childhood should include fun, some young people, both 9 and 12-year-olds, nostalgically recalled past time as more fun than present time, especially at school. They found that school now encompassed harder work and more time spent on it. Fun could be in class with teachers, but especially at break-times with other children.

Dulal:	You get a lot more fun then [i.e. when younger]; and you don't get that now except at dinner-time.
Aisha:	And you get three play-times [i.e. in the past].
Dulal:	More play-times, we want more play-times!

Interviewer: What about you?
Nasma: I liked it better then, it was choosing all day . . .
Aisha: In the afternoons, he [supply teacher who takes the class on Fridays] lets us play games on Fridays. We have fun with him, cos in the morning we did work with him and then in the afternoon we played games.
                  (East Primary School, Year 5, group discussion)

These young people described the school regime as shaping their experience. In particular, they noted the virtues of their supply teacher. The children thought their class teacher was overstrict. He knew he ran a strict regime and I heard him on several occasions explain to the class why: there was so much work to get through this year (in preparation for SATS next year).

Interviewer: What's it like being a child?
Kim: Fun!
Interviewer: And is life fun now?
Kim: No.
Interviewer: Because?
Kim: Not as much, because you don't really get as much time to have fun, do you?
Jackie: You've got all your homework.
Interviewer: So is life tougher this year?
Kim: Yes.
Jackie: Yes. Last year we had about five pieces of [home]work a week and now it's two every day. It's double. And you can't go out and play because you've got your homework.
                  (North Secondary School, Year 8)

School made increasing demands on time as children get older. Kim identified shortage of time and Jackie took up the point – homework takes up time which otherwise could be used for play.

Commonality and difference

There is far more common ground than difference in young people's accounts. The common points are as follows: adults control their lives, but this is how it should be; parents must have authority over children and so must teachers. For childhood is a period of time when you learn, morally and substantively. Parents' authority at home is based on their protection and teaching functions, and school authority is based on teachers' remit. But early childhood at school is easier and more fun than later on, when life gets harder, with more work and less play. Though at school some teachers are unjust, angry and disrespectful, school is enjoyable, a place to learn and interact with friends.

Normatively, they described childhood as a good time, protected and provided for and with opportunities – not to be repeated in adulthood – for experience and learning. Most experienced their childhood in line with these norms. A small minority were inadequately cared for by parents, or faced family problems greater than they felt able to cope with. For those growing up in some Islamic families, especially boys, childhood was hard, because so much had to be fitted in (school, mosque and home duties), but it was nevertheless a good time because the learning activities of childhood were an important basis for the future and experienced as worthwhile now.

Constituting childhood – a note on method

How do young people constitute childhood and how can older people access the processes whereby they do it? In the Childhood Study, I listened and talked with young people in pairs, as individuals and in groups (at East and North Primary Schools and North Secondary School). I started with pairs and when I began to listen to the tapes as I transcribed them and then studied the transcripts, I learned that these conversations are social processes: components of how young people together constitute childhood. Between them they give meaning to 'childhood'.[2] I gathered they had discussed these issues before I elicited them, because their ideas were clearly worked out and clearly expressed; several also told me that one of the functions of friends and the child group more generally is as a forum for discussion of issues that concern them. Thus listening to young people's conversations gives one access to one of the ways in which they line up, confirm, modify and develop their ideas about, in this case, childhood (Smith 1999: 114–19). Probably also the relatively formal character of the research conversations allowed for fuller development of ideas than might always be the case in their own informal conversations. Usually we had an undisturbed period of time, long enough to develop topics; I was there to give each person a chance, to suggest topics, to elicit clarification and detail; they in turn mostly accepted and used the character of the occasion.

In the individual interviews I carried out next, I asked people to tell me about their daily lives and reflect on issues arising. During these interviews, I was of course trying to show my felt sympathy for their story, and I tried to let it be told as the person wished. Reading the transcripts, I became aware that the situation – one young person talking to an older person – resulted in distinctive data compared to pairs and groups. Many of these interviews provided more intense, personal, in some cases distressed, accounts of their own experience. An example of this kind of interview is given by Stuart (p. 83).

Finally I carried out group sessions with four or five people. As with the pairs, there was discussion, swapping of experience and development of themes. These were very jolly sessions: by then they knew me quite well; there were more sparks between them because there were more people to spark off; within the group they recognized their commonality – their common experience and common responses to it. Again, as with the pairs, I would not want to argue that these groups constituted childhood through the discussion, more that they provided a semi-structured forum for developing ideas – and for giving me access to these processes. In the next section, the first two excerpts help to explain these points.

Children as a minority social group

In talking about the social status of childhood, young people support the thesis that childhood is a minority social status. This is not a phrase they use, but it is what they mean. All their accounts point to inequalities between their status and that of adults, and to commonalities between them in their childhood status. They identify power as lying with adults, and regard themselves as dependants who have to obey.

My argument for the idea of children as a minority social group, built up from listening to children and reflecting on their accounts and on their circumstances, also builds on that of socialist feminists, who regard the oppression of women as shaped not only by class (in the Marxist sense – a group's relationship to the economic order) but by gender assignment, as well as by ethnicity; the task then is to develop accounts of these differing types of oppression and of the relations between them (Jaggar 1983: 134). In the case of children, the argument is that children's lives are shaped by the generationing processes specific to various societies, as well as by gender, class and ethnicity; important in these generationing processes is legal designation by age; legally under-18s are 'under age' and less than equal citizens (Saporiti and Sgritta 1990: 1–6). While, as noted above, much of young people's discourse emphasizes the positive sides of childhood, they also note its difficulties, and some say their days are overly controlled by adults, both at home and, especially, at school. As suggested in Chapter 6, most think their protection and provision rights are generally honoured, but that their participation rights are less well and less consistently respected.

I describe here how young people demonstrate their understanding that they belong to a social group which is subordinate to adulthood and derives the processes through which it is constituted and restructured from its relations with adulthood.

A common domain of childhood

> The social construction of reality is precisely that of creating a world we have in common.
>
> (Smith 1988: 125)

Young people indicate that they inhabit a common domain – as children, under the supervision, control and protection of adults. The research conversations show that they share experiences, and recognize and endorse others' experiences; they identify social realities that are common to them in their status as children. This recognition, endorsement and identification constitutes one means whereby they structure their childhoods.

That they share a world in common is very clear to them at school. Their sense of shared social positioning and experience were demonstrated, for instance, through discussions between groups of 9-year-olds about the merits and demerits of school, changes they would like to see and how school now compared to school when they were younger. For instance, at one point, a group of five began to construct their idea of a good school day. Their voices were indistinguishable, but all contributed.

> I think we should have more art. Monday, Tuesday, Wednesday, Thursday, Friday, the whole week.
>
> *Interviewer*: What do you like about it [art]?
>
> You get to do painting and drawing and pens and stuff.
> It's fun. You don't have to do writing.
> The whole class likes it.
> I love art, you can do detail and draw and everything, and lovely sketches and that.
> Everyday we should do –
> 9–10: Art.
> 11–12: sketching.
> Half an hour handwriting.
> Dinner time.
> Afternoon: 1–2 painting.
> 2–3.
> And no homework.
>
> *Interviewer*: Yes, and at the end of the day?
>
> And read a book.
> No, play a game.
> No, have a story.
> Computer.
> And no homework.
>
> (East Primary School, Year 5 group)

These 9-year-olds knew this was creative fantasy – they had accepted the reality of the National Curriculum and homework guidelines – but they were purposefully constructing a day based on what they enjoyed, as a counter to the regime they actually experienced. Their quick-fire construction of this vision, each suggestion building on the previous one, shows how much they were in tune with each other.

On the general topic, bad things about school, another group discussed the 'sanction room' system, whereby children who transgressed rules missed play at break-time, and instead were confined in a room with a teacher.

	You get sent there at dinner-time and play-time.
Interviewer:	Who sends you there?
	The teacher.
Interviewer:	I've not seen this happen while I've been here. Why do people get sent there?
	If you talk in assembly, if you don't do your work.
	If you don't bring your homework book.
Interviewer:	How long do you spend in there?
	The whole play-time.
Interviewer:	Has that happened to any of you this term?
	Jack [he is one of this group].
Interviewer:	So what are the wicked things you do, Jack – talk in assembly?
Jack:	If people are cruel, I beat people up.
Interviewer:	Do you sometimes?
Jack:	If I'm in the mood.
Interviewer:	And are there teachers in this sanction room?
	Yes, they take it in turns. They write your name in the book, and if your name's in the book three times, your parents have to come in.
Interviewer:	Is it a good system or not?
	No [all say this].
	It's bad.
Interviewer:	What's wrong with it?
	If they tell my parents, they'll beat me up.
Interviewer:	Do they?
	If I've been in the sanction room three times, my Dad won't beat me up. But my Mum will.
Interviewer:	When you say, 'beat me up', what would she actually do?
	Slap me on my back, or on my face.
	If I was in the sanction room, I'd tell my parents and my parents would just tell me off.
	Mine would hit me.

Interviewer: What would be a better system?
Give them three more chances and then –
Ten more chances [laughter].
And they'd [teachers] get more fed up with them [children] and leave and then we'd get nicer teachers [laughter].
(East Primary School, Year 5 group)

These young people demonstrated their joint awareness of moral issues involved in this form of punishment. Punishment at school carried over into the home, for teachers could draw parents into the episode. Under UK law, schools may no longer hit children, but parents may; their children were thus exposed to a system whereby adults – across school and home – controlled them. From the young people's point of view, a better procedure would be give children more chances; children should not be written off as problems. With a leap of creativity, the last speaker shows how this procedure might get rid of punitive teachers. Again, the speed of this conversation (which cannot be shown on paper) and the movement of ideas across the comments and suggestions (which can perhaps be discerned), indicates young people's acquired understanding of their points of view as children in contradistinction to adults'.

As children in relation to parents, young people also share a world in common. Through conversations at school, they provide solidarity with others who belong to the relational category child.

Samera: Yeah, if someone is feeling down, you can always tell they're down. You know something's wrong.

Jayda: They say, What's wrong? And you say, Oh, nothing. And they say, I know something's wrong. And then they just tell you [laughter of recognition].

Interviewer: So talking to each other – [it's] a relief?

Jayda: Yes.

Interviewer: Can you help each other in other ways: if something very wrong is happening?

Samera: It depends on the situation, but usually we can.

Jayda: If it's something really family and really private, you sometimes can't let it out, even to your best, best friends. But if it's something that happens once, or maybe just once more then maybe you can tell somebody.
(East Mixed Secondary School, Year 8 girls' group)

These girls gave as an example a girl in their group who needed to talk a lot about her situation; she felt torn between her fostering family and her own mother, whom she saw weekly. They were very familiar with her situation, and indicated that they frequently listened to the updates, sympathized and made suggestions.

Gender is important in confiding. Both girls and boys referred mainly to same-sex friends as confidants, but while some girls and boys aged 9 and girls aged 12 also identified their mothers, 12-year-old boys mostly said they confided, not in mothers but in male cousins, mates and older brothers: 'cos there's girls' things and boys' things' (East Mixed Secondary School, Year 8)

> *Nazidual*:   The best thing [about having mates] is that you can talk to them whenever you've got problems. You just phone them up and talk to them about what you did or can do.
> *Interviewer*: Is that different from how you can talk with your family?
> *Ferdous*:   Yes, because, like, to your family you can't talk about girls and everything, but to your friends you can talk about girls more.
>
> (East Mixed Secondary School, Year 8)

Most of the Asian young people were particularly well placed here. They tended to have well maintained extended family relationships, and thus access to 'girl cousins' and 'boy cousins' both locally, and, by phone, in other parts of the UK.

Sibling solidarity

Solidarity between sibs in dealing with adult-ordered social domains is a feature of stories written for children.[3] Personal experience suggests that sibs do make common cause in face of parental edicts. Research evidence, including mine, is sparse. Some of the 'Asian' children, who had many sibs and cousins living nearby, did talk about their sense of commonality in relation to adult members of their extended families. In general, though, children tended to talk in individual terms, to express both affection for sibs and differences in outlook and behaviour, and rivalry – for space, use of computer, privileges and rights. Perhaps when thinking about home life, young people conceptualize themselves in their individual relations across the generations, rather than, as at school, as members of a social group which acts in tension with the social group teachers. Researchers' own assumptions and research questions will also influence their data. Traditionally, studies have focused on individual relationships between sibs and between sibs and parents, rather than on children's social group solidarities in relation to parents. Research which studies variations in child–parent relations also points to consequent variation in sibs' relations with each other.[4]

Common cause in school

Research with children at school shows clearly that they make common cause in relation to teachers in class-time, in the playground, and as classmates. Discussions among young people at school are an important means whereby they constitute schoolchildren and teachers as distinctive groups. The merits and demerits of teachers are an endless topic for discussion, with emphasis on the relational (see also Chapter 6: 98). Girls at East Mixed Secondary School explained that some teachers were more in tune with them than others. Their English teacher understands them, knows they like a bit of fun – makes jokes during class, 'takes the mick'. Bad teachers are those who tell them not to talk to each other, don't understand that some young people like talking while they work and do better when they are talking. Their comments, at various points in the conversation, demonstrate their shared experience and understanding:

> Some people like being quiet or just whispering. Some people like making jokes when they're working, but most teachers just expect you to get on with it.

> Yeah, we know it's like for our own good to work quietly, but they have to understand and do different things.

> I don't know why, but the work becomes harder when you are quiet. But in English we can like relax a bit and like we can always understand the work and do it a bit quicker than we would usually do in these [other] subjects. . . .

> And you can like ask each other what to do, but like in some subjects you can't and you have to ask the teacher every time . . .

> I think the English teacher understands us, he knows how we feel and what we like to do and what we don't like to do and how long it takes us and everything . . .

> I think they shouldn't forget that we can't always understand what they are saying straight away. They shouldn't expect us to be quiet all the time. You learn from different things.
>
> (East Mixed Secondary School, four Year 8 girls)

While accepting their own minority status, as people who are less competent than their teachers, these girls are asking teachers for sympathy, tolerance and respectful behaviour. They are also pointing to a gap between some teachers' understandings and theirs. Some teachers think students should work as isolated individuals; these girls propose learning as a group activity – with jokes to keep you going and mutual help and support.

Making common cause in the playground is also critical for well-being. Playground environments may be indifferent or hostile to children's interests. The social and physical characteristics of playground commonly facilitate bullying. Children have to spend time there, and cannot control whom they interact with in the small spaces often provided. Small spaces also facilitate accidents. Children help each other face up to bullies, and care for those who feel ill or have an accident (see also Chapter 5). One factor that may reduce the incidence of bullying and accidents is spacious play-space, where children can spread out and escape each other; another is adequate adult supervision and/or provision of group activities.[5] Making and keeping friends, however defined, is crucial to young people's welfare at school, as defence, support, enabling (cf. Sluckin 1981). Five-year-olds at Greenstreet were quite clear about this. You need people to play with you, so that you are not left out and isolated; as a pair or group, you are less likely, than as a person standing alone, to be knocked over.

> *Ralph*: I don't like playing games if it's with people who hate me.
> *Chris*: I play with them even though they're not my friends. People hate me but I still play with them.
> *Bob*: And not playing with anybody. Because it's not very nice. And I don't like looking round for people and them knocking me over.
>
> (Mayall 1994: 59)

Demonstrations of solidarity were given by 9-year-old girls (at North Primary) who were being bullied by one particularly troublesome boy. They would set off for the playground with arms round each other, told me how they had jointly fought the boy, and had accompanied each other to the headteacher to sort out the problem.

Having at least one person on whom you can rely is important for managing difficult experiences at school:

> [The topic being discussed is ways in which people can make childhood better.]
>
> *Nasra*: If you meet someone and you really like that person and they be your friend for six years. [When I was in nursery] I used always to cry in the dinner hall and I didn't have any lunch and then we were in reception and she came and said, 'I haven't got no one – will you be my friend?' And I said, 'OK then'. So then we started to be friends. And I told her all my life story, and she told me her story and we started to be friends.
>
> *Interviewer*: So being friends is very important to you.
>
> *Nasra*: Yes, and in the playground you shouldn't be nasty. If someone falls down, me and P [her friend] run and say, What – ? And the person who fell down, we help them and then we have lots of friendships. That happened to Leila, and she fell down and we said, 'What's your name?

What happened to you?' And then we bumped into her again and we made friends.

(East Primary School, Year 5)

These friendships are important also, of course, not just as defence, but to provide playmates. This girl and her friend later detailed to me the games they played together – some of those passed down through the generations and listed by Iona and Peter Opie (1969). Iona Opie (1993) documented in one playground the social groupings of play; boys' games are particularly intense, aggressive and active, whereas girls' play is more leisurely, and they shift from one game to another instantly and easily. She confirms the point made in the excerpt above: that girls tend to interest themselves in other people, enjoy talking and are hospitable and helpful in the playground.

Another feature of children's social solidarity is their loyalty to their class – the group who go through the school years together. In the Childhood Study, I observed many instances in class-time of children supporting and helping their colleagues. For instance, in the North Year 5 class, one boy was way behind most of the others in maths, and at the end of one session he was still working on a problem; others, not his particular friends, gathered round his desk, in order to make a point of praising his achievements so far. A second example: one of the brightest boys, who happened to be sitting next to one of the slowest boys, spotted his difficulties in understanding the allotted task and helped him with it. A third example: people took me to the wall where poems and drawings were displayed and draw attention to the work of others in their class, as well as their own. A fourth example was a session enabled by the teacher: when one boy had been bullying a girl in the playground, she asked the whole class to listen while each put their case and then encouraged a whole class discussion of the moral issues; their engagement with the discussion suggests their strong feelings about dealing with anti-social behaviour in their class.

Facing up to life

Gender solidarity is important in group support. For instance, a friendship group of five girls provided evidence of the importance to them of their group membership. Three of them came from Asian Muslim families, one from Africa and one from a southern European country. They were all keen to speak, though the European girl spoke less good English and the others helped her. They knew each other well, and each others' stories, and often filled in bits a speaker had omitted or not made clear enough, and added in bits from their own history. They said for them the best thing about school was their friends. 'Because if it wasn't for school, we wouldn't know each other. We wouldn't have that company.' Outside school, the Muslim girls mixed only with the extended family. School provided contact with girls of other religions and backgrounds and a forum for discussion and support. During the research conversation with me, I raised the issue of their futures. The three Muslim girls (Hannaa, Madiha and Aleya) started off:

Interviewer: Have you thought about your futures?

Hannaa: Sometimes your parents plan it.

Madiha: Me and my friend have decided: we're going to do a seven-year course and be doctors.

Interviewer: You've decided.

Madiha: Yes.

Aleya: I don't know, but after this school, I'll go to college and do whatever course I choose.

Hannaa: I'm going to go to college and do a two-year course for nursery nurse. Or be a teacher.

Interviewer: So your family isn't expecting you to get married and have children?

Hannaa: I don't know.

Interviewer: They don't talk about that?

Hannaa: My Mum's always teasing me and saying, 'You've got a boyfriend, you're going to get married' [joint laughter and 'Yeah'].

Aleya: In my family, my [elder] sisters didn't do nothing. [inaudible bit] And my brother-in-law found her her husband. And he works till twelve o'clock at night.

Interviewer: So your parents – they don't say it's obvious you have to get married? Cos some of the 9-year-olds did say that.

Aleya: Sometimes I get told off like, and my mother says, if I'm cleaning something and I don't clean the dishes properly, she says, 'When you get married you – '

Hannaa: Yes, they say, 'When you get married, would you do that, would you do this?'

Aleya: In my family they go behind your back [i.e. arranging marriages].

Jo [the girl from Africa]: I'm thinking of going to a music college, or a drama, acting college. And my Mum's registered me for a college. And my Mum sometimes says, 'Are you going to get married?' and I say, 'No'. Because I hate boys. I'm never going to get married. [More here about going to acting school on Saturdays now.]

Paula [the girl from Europe]: I want to be a lawyer.

Interviewer: Right. Why do you want to do that?

Paula: I don't know. I don't think you have to be very good in [inaudible] to be a lawyer . . . Or if I'm not a lawyer, I want to be a teacher, of babies.

Hannaa: I don't know. My Mum and my brother say I'd be good to be a nurse. I don't know what I'm going to be. But I ain't sure. I don't know yet.

Interviewer: Is there anything you want to do?

Hannaa: I want to be a nurse. But I don't know yet.

Jo: Do you want to get married, Hannaa?

Hannaa: I don't know.

Jo: I'm not. I don't want to get married.

Hannaa: In our family you get arranged marriages.

Madiha: My sister's going to get married in a few days time. When she's finished uni . . .

Hannaa: It's like when we're up to 18 or 19, your parents start looking for a partner. And you won't know about it until they, like, tell you.

Aleya: Isn't it strange sometimes. They like go behind your back.

Madiha: Yes.

Hannaa: My brother's 17, he's going to get married when he's 19. He's only got two years left.

Jo: He's only got two years left to parteee!

[More here about how various relatives have gone to Bangladesh to seek partners for older sibs.]

Hannaa: It's like their acting like you're 13! [more laughter.]

(East Mixed Secondary School, Year 8)

In this conversation these girls gave recognition to each other's situation and family traditions, while also chipping in with comments, and other points of view, expressed not aggressively but responsively and sympathetically. There was a good deal of joint laughter during this 40-minute group research conversation; these were topics they had discussed before, and they were sharing the opportunity provided in this conversation for airing, though with a light touch, the seriousness of the issues they faced. The start of this snatch of conversation already introduced the issue of parental control over girls' futures ('Sometimes your parents plan it'). But then Madiha made a firm statement of her plans for her seven-year college future; this was followed by the more conformist vision of the other two – for a short college course. These girls' expressions of worry and powerlessness, about the likelihood that their parents will arrange a marriage for them, were enabled by the way in which others in the group confirmed what they said, or presented alternative scenarios. They all recognized family traditions on marriage as enduring, but they also knew – as shown in this and other accounts by Muslim girls – that some parents wanted girls to do well at school and go to college, even to work in a career for a year or two, before getting married. The conversation continued (after this excerpt) with examples where parents and other relatives had looked for a partner in Bangladesh. And Jo made her point directly here: ' Shouldn't you choose your own partner, like?' and Aleya replied: 'It's much better, cos then you get to know them.' Sympathetic laughter followed.

In sum, young people's accounts show that they share a common domain in relation to adults. Through friendships and discussions they construct group solidarity which enables them to deal with school and with issues at home. This solidarity helps them analyse and come to terms with their social situation, as minors in both settings; they work through issues, and support each other.

Play

I have given a separate section to this topic, because play features so promin-ently in young people's accounts of childhood, because their accounts are distinctive (compared to adults') and because what they say about it places play firmly within their understanding of child–adult relations.

Adult views of play

Of course, play as a topic for study has traditionally belonged to psycholo-gists and biologists, just as children have (Bruner *et al.* 1976; Sutton-Smith 1979; Hutt *et al.* 1989). Adults in these disciplines have been interested in the functions of play, its usefulness in developmental terms, and in children's 'needs' for play; but they have not generally consulted children. I have found Huizinga's historical and sociological approach useful towards understanding my conversations with children. On the basis of his vast knowledge of human cultures, he argues that most studies of play ignore what play is in itself and what it means for the player (1949: 2–3). The essential quality of play is that it is fun; and once we say that we acknow-ledge that there are active minds engaged in the play. Summarizing his initial discussion he says:

> [Play is] a free activity standing quite consciously outside 'ordinary' life as being 'not serious' but at the same time absorbing the player intensely and utterly. It is an activity connected with no material interest and no profit can be gained by it. It proceeds within its own proper boundaries of time and space according to fixed rules and in an orderly

manner. It promotes the formation of social groupings which tend to surround themselves with secrecy and to stress their difference from the common world by disguise or other means.

(Huizinga 1949: 13)

Huizinga is not interested in children, but he notes that his definition of play can cover animals, children and adults, and sees it as a fundamental category in life (1949: 28). Since his time, the new social studies of childhood have foregrounded children as active participants in constructing their lives. Scholars have argued that in their play they may be seen as acquiring and working up their identities and so engaging in the politics of the playground (James 1998: 103; see also Sluckin 1981). In this adult vision, play is not separate from life, from the mainstream of culture; play has a developmental and social function: performance in play is engagement with real life.

Young people's accounts of play

As I have noted, young people described play as a defining feature of child-hood, in contrast to adulthood, and play is one of the things children do in 'free time' – which they define as time out of adult control. Though young people rarely used formal rights language, they did talk about their 'right' to play, in line with the CRC:

Article 31: States parties recognise the right of the child to rest and leisure, to engage in play and recreational activities appropriate to the age of the child and to participate freely in cultural life and the arts.

(United Nations 1989)

Play is one of the things children do and do well – unlike adults who do not play, are bad at it, and are too busy with, or worn out by, their heavy responsibilities.[6]

Interviewer: Are you children ever?
Fariah: Sometimes, cos you go out to play, and then you're children.
Interviewer: Adults don't play?
Fariah: No.

(East Mixed Secondary School, Year 8 girl)

Robert: Adults are a bit boring . . . they don't really play football or nothing like that . . . They just go to work most of the time, and when they come home they just want their dinner and then sleep afterwards.

(East Mixed Secondary School, Year 8)

This girl associates childhood with imaginative play, but also with absence of major responsibility:

> *Yasmina*: Well, we've moved on from being a child, because we don't play games like mummies and daddies anymore. But I do still state myself as a child because I'm not grown up. Because I'm not working, um, I'm not really taking care of children like adults would do.
>
> (North Secondary School, Year 8)

Play is fun. It comprises the elements adult observers have commonly noted: pretend or fantasy play, singing, clapping and dancing games, enacting well-known stories, sports with formal rules (football), learning and passing on traditional playground games. Young people described playing as, usually, a social event, with two or more people, but one person could engage in fantasy play.

> *Lingi*: Because it's as if you can imagine anything. You can imagine you can do anything. You can pretend to be magic. You don't have to be ordinary. It's not really magic. Like Star Wars – you can pretend you can do things you can't really do – like in the future. They have machines that can do anything.
>
> (aged 8)

Play is a break from the adult-ordered day:

> *Interviewer*: What are the best things about playing?
> *Luke*: It's our free time, from school, teaching, reading and homework.
> *Colin*: And my Mum used to say I was really tired after school and I needed a holiday. And we've got one today [an Inset day].
> *Luke*: It's our time, when we do what we like, more or less.
> *Interviewer*: What do you mean: more or less?
> *Luke*: Teachers don't let us do all of it, like violence. Or play football, except in the football cage.
>
> (aged 8)

Friends and play get top ratings in discussions about the merits of school. Group discussions with 9-year-olds at East and North Schools point to this. Asked to list the best things about school (unprompted), all but two of the 11 groups named play, play-time and friends first off; the other two groups started off with the formal curriculum, and later moved on to play and friends. Sports clubs, games and PE classes also featured strongly in these discussions. Groups regretted there was less time now for play than in earlier years (one less play-time).

However, (as noted earlier, p. 127) at school, even at play-time, the physical and social environment is controlled by adult planners and school staff; teachers call you in to class just as you have established a game; some games are banned, as Luke notes above; use of climbing frames may be restricted; and grassed areas may be out of bounds in wet weather.

Those young people whose homes provided a reasonable amount of space argued that playing was better at home than at school; they had more time there out of direct adult control, and adults interfered less.

Interviewer: How is play different from ordinary life?
Alicia: It's more fun than being taught. But it's not as much fun as playing at home, because at school you're not allowed to do many things.

(6 years)

I would argue, therefore, that the high value young people put on free time, play and fun relates to the predominant character of their days: lived under adult control and supervision. Like Huizinga, they propose play as time out of ordinary life which is absorbing and delightful; in their examples they repeat his points about games having (arbitrary) rules, about the players maintaining social boundaries around their play. Young people do not refer to a developmental need for play (as learning) but they do refer to their need for a break from the adult-ordered day; and for them the function of play is to enable them to experience delight and fun, usually, but not necessarily, in company with friends.[7]

Discussion: towards a child standpoint?

What contributions do discussion of data in this chapter make to developing the notion of a child standpoint?

Childhood as a relational category

My reading of these London young people's accounts is that they share a common domain of childhood, which they experience positively, as a distinctive period of life. Childhood is enjoyable, a time of protection and provision, of privilege and fun, and a time when one learns essential things for the future. They highly value 'free time', especially for the opportunities it gives to step aside from ordinary life into the world of play. Childhood is a status to be made the most of while it lasts.

Common to them, too, is their identification of a central problem arising through their subordinate position in child–adult relations, that they have little part in decision-making. They accept obedience as a relational feature of childhood, but it can be irksome if their participation rights are not respected. They accept this lack as a natural though bad feature of school life, but are more critical about child–parent relations, even where they have absorbed a clear parental edict that children must obey parents.

I argue that the young people studied are implicitly and in some cases explicitly defining themselves as a social group, where young people recognize each other's circumstances and problems with child–adult relations both now and for the future, and offer each other sympathy, support and suggestions. They are, notably, socially aware. Their views are pragmatic; they take childhood as they find it, enjoying the good parts and coping with the downsides. They are people who have acquired over time the ability and knowledge to face up to the social conditions of their lives, to think about them and to make such modifications as are possible. Their accounts of their experiences encompass understandings of their social status, and its relation to the social status adulthood. They indicate both knowledge and critical capacity. Not only do they understand the impacts of adult agendas on their own lives, they also understand that those adults with whom they have contact – that is, mainly, parents and teachers – live lives not entirely of their own making or under their own control.

These commonalities override detail of gender, ethnicity and age. The points they make concern the generational relations of childhood with adulthood. The essential relationship – between the status with acknowledged authority and their own subordinate status – is recognized by 5-year-olds and continues on, even into the teenage years (defined by young people as starting at 13). Though some of the younger ones think secondary school students and/or teenagers have more power to choose, and though some of the older ones also think so, they find that the essentials of the child–adult relationship have not changed.

Towards a child standpoint

People's experiences vary according to their position in the socioeconomic hierarchy; there is no one disinterested, impartial value-free perspective. In order to give a full and multi-faceted account of how the social order works, we must take account of childhood experience alongside those of women and of men. Young people's accounts of childhood are rooted in their immediate socially situated experiences, unique to childhoods now.

Dorothy Smith (1988: 80) follows Marx in arguing that it is through studying the daily social activities and relations of those outside the relations of ruling that one can make clear how the social system is put together, reproduced and transformed. Women's experiences are important because they lay bare the basic organization that is taken for granted by the ruling class. Accounts of women's experiences and lives fill in gaps and areas neglected in mainstream, or malestream accounts. Smith's argument on the gendered relations of ruling can be harnessed to consider childhood as structured through the generational order.

As discussed in Chapter 2 (p. 24), the two social statuses, defined by gender (women) and generation (children) are not, of course, comparable in all respects (see Oakley 1994). Women's relationships, at least in feminism, are structured by gender, children's by intersections of generation and gender.[8] But women and children are both subject to patriarchy; those in power regard both groups as social problems; both suffer from denial of their rights; both groups find it hard to make their points of view heard and respected. So it is important to develop a specific child standpoint. To do this, we have to consider young people's experiences and knowledge in relation to the ideologies, policies and practices which organize their lives through the relations of ruling (Smith 1988: 97). This means taking account of the intersections of generation and gender in the key arenas of young people's daily lives. It means considering commonalities (and diversity) in children's accounts, as constructed at intersections of agency and structure. We can work outwards from what we find.

Children in UK studies tell us of intense mother–child relations, of child-hoods characterized by protection and social exclusion. Underpinning these experiences is a specific kind of family life, structured through social pol-icies ensuring the gendered adult division of labour, built on psychological understandings of 'the family', 'mothering' and 'childhood'. It is because the numerical majority are subordinated to the dominant minority (paid workers) that children – escorted by women – are pushed to the margins of streets and into their homes. Childhoods are lived in specific ways in the interests of the workings of an adult-oriented society, and the lives and fortunes of children and women are tied together in specific ways in that society.

Similarly, in the other main arena of UK childhoods, the state education system, young people experience the neglect and rejection of their particip-ation rights. These experiences relate to wider and long-held views that state-educated children are to be trained for such work as the state requires of them. Furthermore, as socialization projects, their own views are irrelevant to the education project, which works in the socioeconomic interest of the state (Young and Whitty 1977; Meighan and Siraj-Blatchford 1997). Through shaping up experiences, for instance of homework, with its implica-tions for child–mother relations and for children's time-use, and through moving back and forth between those experiences and the social policies that underpin them, one can begin to explain those experiences, and pro-vide a commentary on the social policies that control them.

More generally, young people's accounts of their daily lives provide a commentary on traditions and trends in adult thought. Psychology has traditionally emphasized children as becomings and childhood as preparation. Sociologists of childhood, in seeking to challenge these notions, currently stress the present tense of childhood and children as agents, their participation in constructing their own lives and their relationships with family and friends. But young people themselves explain that they take account of both being and becoming during their daily interactions. Social setting is important here: at school they struggle to maintain agency in the here-and-now in a future-oriented regime; at home interactive agency in the here-and-now is a central enterprise. More generally, young people present themselves as people (beings), active in the structuring of their lives, and they regard some present-day activities as valuable for the future and some for the present. Thus they link together the present and the future.

Like women in relation to male-structured social institutions, children in relation to adult-ordered social institutions are 'valuable strangers' (Harding 1991: 124). Through paying attention to them, we may consider the degree of 'fit' between the social order and their experiences and understandings.

A key example here is the implications of traffic-danger and stranger-danger for childhood. As many adults note, the rights of children to explore give way to the protection of children in their homes. But young people provide a unique and forceful commentary on this protection: its damaging effects on child–parent relations. Constantly having to ask permission, having to negotiate where one can go, when, with whom and for how long is experienced as irksome and conflictual. Their experience exposes fault-lines in social norms for childhood.

Perhaps the moral status of childhood provides the most dramatic instance of misfit between the adult structuring of childhood and young people's own knowledge and experience (Chapters 4 and 6). Young people find that adults routinely reject or ignore their moral competence, yet they do engage with moral issues. However, to an extent they accept adult orthodoxy, and give themselves little credit for their moral agency. A further twist to this tangle is that adults also expect young people to take moral responsibility, both at home and at school. This adult neglect and indeed conceptual misunderstanding accounts for one of the strongest findings in this and other research, that children find their participation rights are not respected. This misfit between experience and societal concepts has to be explained. Those adults who do see children's moral agency in action – mothers at home – are not socially positioned to make their knowledge known and accepted. Institutions and professionals (such as schools and teachers) are relatively more powerful to promote the notion of child incompetence.

Study of the everyday worlds of childhood experience, like the study of women's experience, serves to ground sociology in daily relations between people, both as individuals and as social groups. Thus young people's definitions of, and high valuing of free time and play must be seen in relation to processes in child–adult relations, and notably to the pervasiveness of adult control. This point not only acts as a counter-balance to psychological understandings of the 'functions' of play, it provides justification for rethinking social policies. Rather than reducing children's free time, we could give serious consideration to planning in free time to children's days, at home, at school and in the times and spaces between.

This is only a beginning of the study of a child standpoint. I am arguing that including young people's knowledge in intersection with adult knowledge is essential in three major tasks. It is an essential journey of discovery: to provide a coherent account of how a constituent social group of the population experience and understand their social positioning. It is essential for working towards a more comprehensive account of how the social order works, and in particular the degree of fit between these valuable strangers' experience and the relations of ruling. And it is essential as a first step towards shifting how adults think about adult–child relations, and towards taking account of young people's experience and knowledge in reshaping the social order. On all counts it is a political enterprise.

8 | Comparing childhoods

Introduction

In this chapter, the daily lives of 9-year-olds in North Primary School, London (Childhood Study) and in a suburb of Jyväskylä, Finland form the starting point for considering how to account for the distinctive characters of these two sorts of childhoods. Rationales for making this comparison are three. A comparison may throw light on one's own society, by drawing attention to or problematizing issues that seem natural or uncontested. Comparison between UK and Finland is useful because the two societies are both welfare states, but are very different in their histories, policies and practices and, in complement, in their understandings of childhood. Third, the Childhood Study was designed alongside a Finnish one carried out by Leena Alanen, so that they could be compared.[1] Leena has made many contributions to this chapter, both on 'facts' and interpretation.

The aim of this chapter is to explore social, economic and cultural mechanisms which generate the daily lives of children, and how these mechanisms differ in the two countries where the study children live. The chapter starts with descriptions of the study children's daily lives, moves on to describe some general patterns in these childhoods and then considers how to account for differences.

Two sorts of childhoods – UK and Finland

Daily lives of 9-year-olds in the two studies

London children

In the UK, both school hours and parental work-hours structure children's daily lives, because social norms assume children will be supervised by an adult. As regards 29 North 9-year-olds (Childhood Study), adults' organization of the day reflects the perceived need to cover the school run at the start and end of the school day. The arrangements they made included: working at home; working part-time; employing an au pair; enlisting another parent or relative to escort or 'mind' the child. In 9 two-parent households traditional UK patterns persisted, with the father out at work and the mother at home (6) or in part-time work (3); in 3 two-parent and 4 one-parent households no one was in paid work; but in 9 two-parent and 3 one-parent households the parents worked full-time. Five of these fathers were step-fathers, some of whom were only sometimes resident. Some, but not all, of the mothers not in paid work had younger children, including babies from these subsequent relationships.

The children attended a school (from 9.00 to 3.30) sited in an inner London suburb at the intersection of two roads; for some of them, their route allowed them to cross on a zebra crossing near the school gate; for others their route meant crossing a road with rush-hour traffic going past. The school is a three-storey Victorian building with asphalt playgrounds, the whole surrounded by a high brick wall; all the children entered through a doorway set in the wall. Apart from school starting and ending times, the door was locked and people could gain entry only after identifying themselves on an answer-phone system.

Only 12 of these 29 children (9 of 17 boys and 3 of 12 girls) went alone or with friends to and from school. The rest were accompanied by an adult or, rarely, an older sib. The scene at the start and end of the day is of children and mothers around the school door; some mothers accompanied their children to the classroom to talk with the class teacher, or to see children's work displayed on the walls.

Though in the 1990s the emphasis in education policy and some practice has shifted to individualism and competition, the school day (in many schools) is characterized by some features persisting from more 'progressive' ideas about education. The teacher in this class modified the demands of the National Curriculum to suit her ideas about pedagogy. The children sat in pairs or groups around a table in a classroom where tables and desks were frequently reorganized, depending on the proposed emphasis – on group or individual work. In general, children talked to each other and worked together. There was little whole-class teaching, and the teacher spent most of the time with groups and individuals. School was the main forum for being with friends, both in class and at break-times.

The whole school (350 children) had a mid-morning break out in the playground – which consequently was crowded and busy. At midday, a school meal was provided (subsidized, with parental contribution), but many of the children brought their own packed lunch. One of the school's three big halls was used for the midday meal.

After school, at 3.30, most of the children went home first, and had something to eat. In most cases an adult was present at home. Some then went out (again mostly escorted) to various activities: mainly sports, arts and drama groups. Six of the 12 girls and 13 of the 17 boys attended one or more session per week in this kind of activity. As to going out unaccompanied, as I indicated in Chapter 6 (p. 103), this was a matter of negotiation, usually for each occasion, with mothers. Three of the 12 girls were allowed only to go to their friend 'next door' and another three said they 'played out' sometimes. Of the 17 boys, two went only to friends' homes, and another 10 said they played out (see also Table 6.1). These children had homework only once a week, to be done over the weekend and handed in on Monday.

Finnish children
Finnish school-age children are expected to manage their daily lives. The 20 9-year-olds (one class at school) lived with one or two parents, all of whom were in paid employment, though some were at home on parental leave or childcare leave, or registered as unemployed.[2] In some cases, their parents had already left for work before they themselves set off for school. Most woke themselves up (with an alarm clock), made their breakfast, assembled their belongings and walked or cycled to school. Most of the journeys were on paths and tracks separated from car traffic, but where a road had to be crossed there were narrowed crossings, lights and 'green men'.

The children live in Jyväskylä, central Finland; and their school is sited in a modern suburb. Unlike the London school, it has no formal boundary wall or fencing. The playgrounds abut the local woods, and anyone can come and go. At play-times, some children play at the edge of the woods, as well as on the main tarmacked playspaces. The school is a one-storey building, with wide corridors with pegs and lockers for the children's belongings – important in a country where big coats and boots are needed to come to school in winter.

The school day for this age-group ran from 8 a.m. to 2 p.m. Judging by my observation of a school day, the regime was relatively formal compared to the UK model. The children each had a desk, arranged in lines and rows, facing forwards to the teacher, who explained topics to the whole class, gave instructions and presented material on a blackboard. The children were meant to work individually (for a similar picture, see Gordon *et al.* 2000: Ch. 5). Finnish teachers are autonomous professionals who may choose their methods; this teacher, judging by her own comments, was perhaps more traditional than some, but during her fieldwork months Leena saw group work in progress every day in some lessons.

The school day, as in the UK, had regular breaks for the children (supervised by an adult), but the teacher could also give the children a break at the end of a work session. So then only some of the school's children would be out in the (very spacious) playground. Towards midday, the children went to a purpose-designed canteen (with attached kitchen), where a free meal was provided.

After school, they went home; most then rang their mother to say they were back, and agreed to do their homework (each weekday) before any other activity. Commonly, they would make themselves a snack and organize their afternoon/early evening – at home alone or with friends, or out and about, at the library or afterschool centre. They varied in how many formal classes or groups they belonged to and attended; some stressed their friendship groups, others pursued their own interests such as playing instruments or sporting activities.

Two kinds of childhood
On the basis of these daily lives, what are the key differences between these two sorts of childhoods?

- The London children are continuously under adult supervision at home and school.
- Their use of public space, unaccompanied by adults, is strictly under parental permission.
- They socialize with peers mainly in each other's homes, but somewhat in the neighbourhood.
- The Finnish children manage their daily lives at home, to school and out of school.
- They have access unaccompanied to neighbourhood facilities.
- They have good opportunities for socializing with peers outside the family.

We can next describe some differing social conditions underlying these differing childhoods.

Some general patterns

Young childhoods
Children mostly base their early childhoods in their parents' households, and so we must describe policies that affect parents' daily lives. Though

welfare states differ in their provisions around childbirth and the first years of childhood, it seems that in most if not all states, gender remains a determinant of women's and their children's lives; in both 'our' countries it is women who take responsibility for childcare (Bryson *et al.* 1994; Sainsbury 1994a). But UK and Finnish provisions for parents and children differ widely, and so, therefore, do young children's daily lives.

In both the UK and Finland, packages of financial benefits and daycare provision are essential if women are to have equal employment opportunities. UK parental leave provisions at the birth of a child are the worst in the European Union; under the Labour government (since 1997) provisions are slowly improving, mainly in response to pressure from the European Union. Currently maternity leave is granted for 40 weeks with payment at 90 per cent of earnings for six weeks and a flat rate for an additional 12 weeks. Parental leave is slowly being introduced to encourage fathers to take part, but so far with no payment attached (*Guardian* Money section, 9 June 2001, p. 11).

There are few state-funded daycare places for under-5s, restricted to those whose mothers are in dire straits.[3] State-funded nursery education places are available for some children aged 3 and 4, mainly part-time – free to parents – but these do not provide daycare which enable mothers to go out to full-time work. A patchwork daycare system (playgroups, minders, nannies, au pairs, relatives, day nurseries) has developed which partially fills these gaps. During the pre-school years of 'my' 9-year-olds, state daycare places were available for only 1–2 per cent of children, and free state nursery education for about one-quarter (almost all part-time places). If their mothers went out to work, they would have used various combinations of daycare, depending on their wealth and local availability.

In the UK, especially since the 1970s, increasing proportions of mothers 'go out to work', mostly part-time. In both countries, the proportion of families headed by one parent has grown in recent years; for the UK it is estimated at 22 per cent in 1995 (Office for National Statistics 1998) and of these over 90 per cent are women; for Finland the proportion in 1998 was 15.8 per cent, of whom again most (88.6 per cent) were women (Kartovaara and Sauli 2000). Figures for 2000 show that in the UK only half as many 'lone mothers' of pre-schoolers do paid work, compared to 'partnered mothers' (Office for National Statistics 2000: Table 4.8). This is attributable to the inadequate supply and high cost of daycare as well as to the extra difficulties a lone mother faces of juggling paid work and childcare. Full-time work is especially difficult for mothers with young children. The figures for partnered and lone mothers even out somewhat when their youngest child is at school. Notably, UK demographic studies do not generally deal with men's employment in relation to their parental status, since men's employment is not affected by parenthood.

So in the pre-school years, UK family policies ensure that children's daily lives are conditioned by individual family circumstances: by constraints on mothers, and by such choices as mothers can make. There are wide variations, built on huge disparities in income and high rates of child poverty – currently at 21 per cent compared to 3.4 per cent in Finland (Micklewright and Stewart 2000). Some children will have mothers in full-time well-paid work, with nannies or au pairs on hand, and will go to playgroup or nursery school part-time from the age of 2 or 3. Others will have mothers working for low pay, paying for daycare at childminders. Most children will spend some or all the day with their mother, for less than a fifth will have a mother in full-time work, and children with lone mothers are especially likely to spend their days mainly with their mother. But from the age of 3 years a large majority of children will attend part-time playgroups (generally at low cost to parents) and/or state nursery schools and classes (free).

In Finland, the state has implemented three measures to support parents and children (Leira 1998), and these somewhat reduce the impact of individual family circumstances on children's experiences. Parental leave for 28 weeks after a child's birth is funded at about 70 per cent of earnings, and most mothers (but few fathers) take it. Beyond those weeks, a childcare allowance, introduced in 1985, pays parents (but only at about 15 per cent of average wages) who wish to care for under-3s at home (Salmi 1996); some municipalities add a homecare allowance to this to increase uptake. Third, the Finnish state (since 1973) requires municipalities to provide daycare on demand, also afterschool services; parents contribute on a means-tested basis. Thus parents have some flexibility and choice in arranging their days. However, the childcare allowance is attractive mainly to low earners or high-earning dual earners. The figures indicate that it is common for parents of over-3s to do paid work; while virtually no under-1s are in daycare, a third of 2-year-olds are, half of 3-year-olds and two-thirds of 5- and 6-year-olds (Kartovaara and Sauli 2000).[4]

There is still a gender gap in parents' employment. Of all under-18s, 86 per cent have a father in employment, and 69 per cent a mother in employment, and mothers' (but not fathers') employment rises with the age of their youngest child, from 51 per cent of mothers of under-2s to 78 per cent of mothers of 13–17-year-olds (Kartovaara and Sauli 2000). Thus in general Finnish children will experience their mother as main caregiver, and many will spend their early years at home with her, but most will have extensive experience of daycare from 3 years.

Schooldays
Just as young childhoods are structured by differing contributions by the state and parents, so too are schooldays.

In the UK, compulsory schooling is from 5 to 16 years. In most parts of the UK, the first school/primary school is for 5 to 10/11 year-olds and secondary school for 11 to 16 (and 17 to 18) year-olds. About 8 per cent of school-age children go to private schools, with higher proportions, especially at secondary level, in some areas (such as London). The education system has become highly centralized since the early 1990s, with a national curriculum and regular tests.

The primary school day generally runs from 9 to 3.30, with a midday meal: school dinner (state-subsidized with contribution from parents) or a packed lunch.

Most schools do not have a sick room and school nurse on site; care for children is provided on an ad hoc basis by teaching and non-teaching staff. Schools sometimes summon mothers to pick up their children if they are ill.

In Finland, compulsory schooling runs from 7 to 16 years, and schools comprise a lower school for the first six years and upper school for the following three years. Virtually all schools are comprehensive (negligible proportions of school-age children go to private schools). In the 1990s, the education system has been decentralized to the municipalities, and they and teachers are responsible for the curriculum.

The school day starts at varying times between 8 and 9 a.m. and its duration lengthens as children get older. For 9-year-olds, it generally ends at about 2 p.m. In Finnish society, the main meal of the day is taken at midday, and both schools and places of work provide this. For school children it is free.

Schools generally have a sickroom for the care of children who fall ill or have an accident, staffed by a school nurse who will be on site for varying periods, depending on municipal decisions and on the geographical location of the school.

Thus the Finnish education system takes fuller responsibility for the care of children while they are at school, both in sickness and in health, than the UK system, which operates an uneasy compromise between state and parental responsibility. On the other hand, the earlier age of compulsory school attendance and the longer school day from age 5 in the UK provide a free daycare service (on one site) earlier than in Finland.[5]

Life outside school
In the UK, it is generally assumed that primary-aged children will be supervised by adults (or older sibs) at all times, though at age 9 some go to and from school unaccompanied. Most return to a home with an adult present. Though some, and especially boys, are allowed 'to play out' with friends, they are commonly accompanied on journeys to parks, out-of-school classes and activities and to friends' homes. In recent years, there has been an expansion in out-of-school services, used mainly by children whose parents

are out at work (Smith and Barker 2000). As discussed in Chapters 4 and 6, parents' concern about traffic danger and stranger danger leads them to restrict their children's use of public space, especially that of girls.

In Finland, the practices of daily life, for both parents and children, encourage school-age children's independence at home and in the neighbourhood. Almost all children are responsible for organizing themselves first thing in the morning, and for travelling to school. They mainly walk or cycle, alone or with friends. After school, children go home on their own or with friends, do their homework and then organize the afternoon and early evening time: with friends outside or at home, attending classes and groups, spending time at the library or afterschool centre. Then parents and children meet at home for an evening meal.

Accounting for difference

How are we to account for the differences between the daily lives of children, living in two welfare states, and between the understandings of childhood that underpin these differing daily lives? During the course of the two studies – in Jyväskylä and London – the researchers (Berry Mayall and Leena Alanen) have considered what factors help explain the differences. They seem to lie in social and material processes over time, including relationships between the state, the family and children, women and children in the divisions of labour, characteristics of the education system. We have separated these out for convenience of discussing them, but they are intricately interlinked. Later we summarize what these analyses tell us about differing models of childhood in the two societies.

The state, the family and children

Deeply rooted traditions provide a basic framework for accounting for difference in childhoods. Within these, we may want to point to differences in the types of welfare state that have developed in the two countries. Critical here are gender issues – which are integral to policies on the family (see below).

In the UK during the long Conservative reign (1979–97), when the children in the Childhood Study were born and growing, longstanding traditions on relationships between the state, family and children were re-emphasized and strengthened through policies designed to emphasize the privacy of 'the family' and its responsibilities for its members. For instance, a 1994 policy statement elaborated four essential duties of government in relation to families: to acknowledge the privacy of the family and parental responsibilities; to ensure that the legal framework underpins family life; to ensure that protection and help is available when families do not provide the support they should; and to support public, voluntary and private bodies which provide practical help to families (Cronin *et al.* 1996: 169). The 1989 Children's Act also emphasized parental responsibility for childcare, with the state as provider and protector where parents failed (Hendrick 1994: Ch. 11). Consonant with these policies was the absence of measures to enable women to combine paid employment with childcare.

Thus state policies played down the generational contract between state and individuals, and played up parental responsibility, with the state having residual functions. Much of this retreat by the state was at the rhetorical level only; the reality was that during those years state policy interventions and neglect led, for instance, to threefold increases in numbers of children in poverty and ever-growing income inequalities (Ennew 1994: 9–11). The inherent conflict between a market-oriented, individualistic approach and respect for rights assumed new prominence within Conservative policies (Oppenheim and Lister 1996: 114–18; Save the Children 1995: 41). The present Labour government, elected in 1997, appears to be continuing with selective, targeted policies on 'families' and 'children's services' rather than with universalist, rights-based policies; universal access and issues of equity remain problematic in the education service (Toynbee and Walker 2001: Chs 1, 3).

The power of history to affect current behaviour can also be seen in state policies specifically directed towards children. As Therborn (1993: 107–9) says, England was the first country to massively abuse children (as labourers in the Industrial Revolution), and the first to take legal measures to protect children; a series of acts thenceforward led to the establishment of institutions devoted to child protection. Voluntary child protection bodies (such as Barnardo's), established in the late nineteenth century in response to massive child poverty and social inequality, were the basis for state childcare services developed through the twentieth century. For a number of complex reasons (Parton 1991), these narrowed their focus almost exclusively to child protection, especially from the 1980s onwards. In England, the protection of children has become key to how children are understood: as vulnerable objects of concern.[6] Protection and to a lesser extent provision remain the linchpins of child institutional practices. The child as citizen – with participation rights – is not enshrined in policy (e.g. James and James 2001).

In Finland, during the early 1980s, diametrically opposed policies were put into legislation, based on earlier practices (Alanen 1996). Policy on child welfare was formalized on universalist principles, grounded on developments aimed at strengthening the welfare state. Though Finland started later (in the 1960s) than Sweden and Denmark on this work, Nordic societies share a social democratic welfare regime/model which is distinctive in key ways: comprehensiveness – the scope of public policy is broad and the state has a larger role vis-à-vis the market and civil society than in most other countries; full employment policy; equality on gender, class, age, ethnicity, religion and region; universality – the right to basic social security benefits in a wide range of life situations and contingencies; high quality benefits – with services provided by professional staff (Kvist 1999: 232). At the heart of the Nordic welfare state is the principle of solidarity – building a consensus state on universalist principles.

Universalist publicly provided social services are key to the Nordic welfare state regimes and are especially highly developed for children and frail elderly people. But though the Nordic social care model 'may be the product of the welfare state and the 1960s, its roots go deeper still, in fact all the way back to the Reformation' (Sipilä 1997: 2). The growth of such services from the 1960s in Finland was based on 'the long-standing ambition to ideologically reform social welfare. The idea was to transform objects [of welfare] into subjects, to move away from forcing people to adapt towards effecting change in society, to fight for civil rights and freedoms' (Sipilä 1997: 3).

This has been a structural approach, whereby the social position of children in society was addressed, through ensuring that their living conditions and the services provided were such that they would not cause children to become problematic 'cases'. During the 1980s, legislation on the principle of the child's best interests was passed to implement these policies. Thus the Finnish state was asserting its generational responsibilities to its youngest citizens, directly, and not just through the medium of the family.

Thus, by contrast with the UK, Finnish social policy has been based on solidaristic principles, stressing both state responsibility for individual people and individuals, including children, as active citizens. A recent summary notes: the state and municipalities have major responsibilities for the well-being of the people; social security is a combination of universal flat-rate benefits for all citizens and earnings-related benefits for paid workers; the basic unit in the provision of social benefits and services is mainly the individual, and not the family; equality of citizens is important: services and opportunities should be given to everyone regardless of their situation (Taskinen 1996).

Traffic danger and stranger danger
Current UK figures for traffic deaths and other death by injury (including 'child abuse') are lower than for any country except Sweden; Finnish figures are slightly higher (UNICEF 2001).[7] Yet protecting children from these dangers is high on UK parental agendas and less so on Finnish ones (it seems). The UNICEF report points to a decline in UK child deaths, and puts it down to increased parental surveillance, safety bought at a price (see Hillman 1993). Finnish parents appear to value children's independent use

of public space, but the Finnish state has almost certainly provided physic-ally safer environments for children than the UK has.

As to 'stranger danger' this seems not to be on Finnish parental agendas. (Indeed in Norway, a country with similar values, and similar death rates, it is alleged that tolerance of accidents is accepted as a necessary corollary of children's independence – Frønes *et al.* 1990: 27.) Apart from models of childhood, it is hard to point convincingly to mechanisms that account for national or cultural difference. Judith Ennew (1986: 181) argues that we need to understand child abuse in the context of two sets of power relations: men/women and adults/children; to the extent that children lack rights, these power relations will impinge particularly hard on them; to the extent that their rights gain greater recognition, child abuse will diminish. Sharon Stephens (1993) agrees that we need to look carefully at mechanisms whereby increased respect for children's material and social welfare and for their rights may decrease not only moral panics on their behalf, but also actual danger to them. A simple and important point is that the abuse of children is more likely among the poor than the wealthy (Parton 1985: 167–9); to the extent that Finland has tackled poverty and income differentials, one might expect lower rates of violence to children.

So perhaps there is less violence to children in Finland than in the UK, but other observers are somewhat sceptical. Alanen and Bardy (1990: 12) express concern about levels of violence towards children. Taskinen (1996: 150) notes that Finland's first report on the CRC to the United Nations in 1994 stressed the need for prosecution of sexual offenders against children. Pringle (1998: 169–73) argues that violence against children in Nordic countries is underreported and unrecognized, and suggests that the absence of well established child protection agencies may partly account for this, whereas in the UK, as noted above, institutional concern for children is long established (Pringle 1998: 104).

Somewhat weakly, perhaps we have to fall back on intersections of these factors to explain differences in children's use of public space.

Gender issues in the division of labour

Gender is a key variable in interrelations between the state, parents and children. The roots of gendered differences within the two societies go way back; and one way of looking at gender in current policy and practice is through grounding understanding in historical processes over a century and more.

As outlined in Chapter 5, social class stratification was well established in mid-nineteenth-century UK society. Well-to-do, middle-class households were models: women at home, running the home and insulated from the rigours of the marketplace; their children were to be protected and nurtured at home and school. This model contrasted with the lives of most children, at work, in poverty, with little or no schooling (Davin 1990).

These established intersections of social class and gender were not seriously challenged in twentieth-century policy; indeed psychological theory (especially from the 1920s onwards) was invoked as justification for the mother–housewife model. The psychological gaze concentrated attention on individual relationships, and the mother as moulder of the young child (Hardyment 1983: Ch. 3). The blueprint for the welfare state – the Beveridge Report (1942) – defined married women, and their children, as dependants of men: 'During marriage most women will not be gainfully employed' (quoted in Wilson 1977: 150). This vision of maternal responsibility and subordination was powerfully endorsed by Bowlby (1953) who emphasized a close continuous relationship between mother and child as necessary for good child development. The notion that defective mother–child relations had long-term adverse effects on children was a powerful tool in the hands of policymakers through the 1950s and onwards; successive governments refused to provide or promote daycare. In the 1980s the Conservative government reinforced, through a number of measures, parental economic responsibility for children, with financial penalties for lone mothers who did not reveal the absent father's identity (Oppenheim and Lister 1996). In the 1990s, however, other factors have led to changes: rising levels of girls' educational qualifications, high costs of living, the rise of lone motherhood have led to mothers returning to work earlier, and this has been enabled by dramatic rises in private provision of daycare.

The general points are first that UK women have been largely excluded, in theory and in practice, from central participation in constructing the welfare state – as citizens, politicians and workers. Second, that childcare was early established as the principal activity of mothers, and it remains mothers' responsibility. Thus the gendered welfare state underlies the specifically UK gendered generational relations within families. Children are tied to mothers in dependence. Nowadays, inconsistent social policies stress mothers' childcare responsibility and paid employment responsibilities, but continued inadequate provision of daycare ensures that part-time work is the solution for many mothers of young children; and this establishes a gendered division of labour between parents; mothers are much more likely than fathers to continue the major responsibility for childcare as the children get older. The ties between children and their mothers therefore become very strong, and it is notable that where parents separate, the children almost always stay with the mother.

The modern Finnish state has developed from a traditional rural patriarchy, with a very small middle class/bourgeoisie until the 1950s. It is estimated that in 1950 half the population was engaged in agriculture or forestry, and men, women and children were employed and understood as workers in the family work order. Though most children attended school from the late nineteenth century, it was made compulsory (from age 7) only in 1921 (Taskinen 1996), and they generally combined family work with school attendance. Within the lifetime of present-day parents and grandparents, the child as worker in the family was an experienced reality.

Traditionally and now women have been regarded as workers. Women have been involved in the construction of the welfare state from the early nineteenth century onwards. The National Project has defined women's mothering activity at home as work (paid in the first three years); and women have never lost participation in the labour market. Whilst in Norway and Sweden there was a period in the 1950s and 1960s when the mother as housewife was a social norm, this was never so in Finland. Thus women have been integrated into society through their participation in the labour market and in politics. (Universal female suffrage was granted in 1906 in Finland compared to 1928 in the UK.) Gender relations between adults can be seen as interacting with generational relations: the provision of education, daycare, health and social services facilitates women's participation in paid work, and this provision also changes children's participation in social life – and thus in the relations between the generations (Alanen 1996).

Finland was industrialized late but rapidly and this has affected the cultural heritage of the welfare state; many elements from an agrarian society have remained, such as strong emphasis on family farms, self-governance and autonomy (Simonen and Kovalainen 1998: 250). This heritage also extends to understandings of childhood and of what children are capable of managing, and, consequently, to adults' everyday practices with children (Alanen 1996).

As noted above, family policies endorse this vision of women as workers both at home and 'at work', by covering the childhood years through benefits and services which enable children and parents to live manageable lives. Parents have the right to take time off 'work' to care for ill children; unpaid, but many employers pay for this (Salmi 1996). It is notable that Finland has not encouraged part-time work, unlike other Nordic countries. The dual-breadwinner family model has been supported not so much by the traditional rural value: dignity through work (though this value is upheld), but more basically because two earners have been, and continue to be, necessary to support a family economy.[8] In the 1950s, the ideology of the home-based wife/mother did have some support, as part of the efforts by cultural elites to modernize Finland after World War II. There were many housewives in the 1950s, taking care of the baby boom children (born 1945–9). But then the birth rate fell, there were more jobs for women, and the gender equality debate of the 1960s put an end to that particular ideological discussion.

As to unpaid domestic work, it seems that whilst Finnish men are not doing more, Finnish women are doing less than they did, probably because such tasks as cleaning, cooking, laundry and childcare are less time-consuming than they were. Not only time-saving gadgets, but Finnish policies on housing, daycare services and meals at work reduce women's work at home. Thus women's rights as citizens somewhat modify the effects of their gender position (Bryson *et al.* 1994).

In terms of the power of psychological discourses on childhood, Finland has been in some respects sited at the edge of Europe. The kindergarten movement was strong at the end of the nineteenth century and kindergartens were established in bigger towns, mainly for children of working women. The kindergarten movement was based on pedagogical theories, and the services were provided as education, not as welfare. The main difference, compared to the UK, is that the urban working class was small in Finland; most industry was in the countryside where resources (wood, water power, the labour force) were sited. Children of the rural working class continued to live very much as rural children; many families worked in small family farms. The class structure was therefore somewhat different, combining agrarian and industrial elements. So psychological knowledge, and kinder-gartens as expression of this, clashed with the actual social and material conditions of women and children. However, in the wake of the 1970s' development of daycare services for pre-schoolers, commentary on psycho-logical issues did emerge into the accompanying debate, which focused not only on the cost, but on the 'proper' place for a young child and his or her mother (Taskinen 1996). More recently, with the growth of psychology as a discipline in Finland, including as an academic discipline (influenced by US/UK ideologies), there has been a move to suggest that the children's independent living styles may be construed as parental deprivation (notably not 'maternal' deprivation!).

National educational projects

The social status of schoolchildren in the two societies nowadays differs (though it is hard to pin down). I suggest the following. In the UK, school-children are positioned as individually responsible for learning what the state prescribes, but within dependent relations with teachers and mothers. They are not citizens, but are preparing for adult citizenship and participa-tion in the workforce. Finnish schoolchildren are understood as citizens of the welfare state. Though their school day may be seen as a top-down teacher–pupil regime, essentially children and teachers are engaged in a joint enterprise through which the children will learn what citizens need to know.

How are we to explain the social status of children at school? A central issue here is how far the establishment of state education systems was and is aimed at building a certain sort of society. For the UK, I noted earlier in Chapter 5 that a thriving private school system used by elites has structured the character of the state system from the start; state schools have never attracted wholehearted support from political elites. Andy Green (1990, 1997: 94–7) argues that Britain has a specific history compared to some other states. In the late nineteenth century, Britain had achieved territorial integrity and stable institutions; it had an established industrial base and an empire. The new education system (established through a series of Acts from 1870) was not designed primarily to help forge a national identity. However, in a society riven with social class differences and conflicts, one aim was to reduce the perceived risk of revolution and, more positively, to integrate the working classes into conformity with middle-class ways of life through monitoring and modifying their morals, health and behaviour.

From the mid-1990s, this vision has clearly underpinned commentary by right-wing and now middle-ground ('New Labour') politicians, who stress the failures of state-educated children to reach prescribed targets. So the education system is structured by the wider societal order, stratified by social class. Responsibility for success and failure attaches to the children and the teachers, rather than to the funding of schools and to the rigid curriculum with its accompanying tests. Children themselves seem to be regarded as objects of the system (doing what they are told) rather than active subjects. Recent government moves to introduce citizenship education into state schools underline the children's non-citizen status; they are to be taught as future citizens (for discussion see Wyness 2000: Ch. 5). As I also suggested in Chapter 5, we have unique intersections of gender and generation in the UK system. The longstanding view that academic achievement relates to mothers' involvement in the school has been taken up with a vengeance; the home–school contract attempts to enforce mothers' cooperation with school agendas, including working with their children on homework assignments.

In general it can be said that the UK education system as currently operationalized emphasizes difference – difference in the quality of children's work – which is mediated by social class (the intake of the school), competition between schools, and input by mothers. So-called 'parental choice' of schools increases difference, as well-to-do parents choose certain schools and avoid others.

By contrast, the compulsory state education service in Finland was established as an important component of a forward-looking nationalism. After the break with Soviet Russia (1917), and a harsh civil war (1918) the Finns had powerful incentives to build a new nation. The aim was, and perhaps still is, to construct a consensus society, with universalist services, based on centralized control of the distribution of resources. For several decades, education was the main 'welfare' service, since Finland was a poor country; other state welfare services developed mainly after World War II. The establishment of compulsory schooling in 1921 formalized existing practice and was based on principles of equal provision and equal opportunity for all. There are very few private schools, and these are mainly ones operating on specific principles (for instance Steiner); they do not pose a threat to the status of the state schools. According to a study of citizenship education in Helsinki and London schools, Finnish schools promote homogeneity and consensus; issues of difference along the dimensions of gender and ethnicity are less fully addressed than in the London schools (Gordon et al. 2000: Chs 2, 3, 9).

Finally, a few general points about the social status of schoolchildren in the two countries. First, what are the prospects for democratic practices in schools? In neither the UK nor Finland are there any legal requirements for schools to establish democratic systems or practices, such as school councils. But whereas in the UK central control over the formal and informal regime has strengthened during the 1990s, in Finland decentralization of decision-making, curricula and other school services perhaps opens up possibilities for democratization. It is not known what is happening in schools, in practice.

A second point is, perhaps, that the divisive features of the UK system can be seen as leading to children being seen as objects rather than subjects, while the Finnish system, with its emphasis on universalist same-quality education for all, may limit children's active engagement with the curriculum, but may paradoxically give children status as people deemed worthy of good quality education; and working with teachers to achieve it.

Perhaps the stakes are too high in both countries for children to be respected as participating citizens at school. The high cost of education services, combined with the possibilities they offer for social engineering, perhaps makes it difficult to recognize children's rights, even in Finland, where otherwise these are respected.

Discussion

This chapter has used comparison with Finland in order to account for London childhoods, and more broadly English ones. In so doing, I find much to admire in Finland and deplore in England. But it must also be noted, that there is not much information from Finnish children on how they experience their childhoods; and no child can simultaneously experience – and evaluate – both kinds of childhood. Further, some Finnish adults argue that some children may suffer parental deprivation and may not enjoy daycare; that they may experience loneliness as a component of their more autonomous childhoods; that they may run risks if traffic calming is inadequate (Leena Alanen, personal communication). English children may derive great happiness from their close relations with parents, especially mothers, and from their protected childhoods; children do express such views. Therefore, the comparison is hedged about with value judgements. After this disclaimer, here are a few final points.

Models of childhood in two societies – a summary

In the UK:

- Children are subsumed under 'family'; policies are targeted at 'families', meaning parents. Parents are essentially regarded as responsible for children's welfare unless unable or unwilling to cope. Children are seen as a cost to parents, and where parents fail, to the state. Universalism is only patchy.
- The social class system ensures that only middle-class children are seen as a potential benefit to the state. Social class/income differences in ways of life persist and have increased from 1979–97. These social divides have supported and promoted a culture of victim-blaming, reduced support for families, privatized services. The private education system ensures that powerful people such as politicians and the wealthy regard state education as inferior for inferior people (see discussion in Chapter 5).
- Children are not productive, not workers, but are in a preparatory stage of life.
- Children are vulnerable, in need of protection and adult supervision.
- Dangers from traffic and strangers justify social exclusion.

In Finland:

- Children are understood as a responsibility of the state (within the National Project); the family is understood as a structural element of the state. Children are less reliant than in the UK on family resources for their well-being and progress.
- Social class and income differentials are not pronounced; services are universalist. Almost all children go to state schools, which provide an even standard of service across the country.
- Children are understood as national capital. Children are productive – as workers at school, just as they were in the former family work order.
- Children are seen as independent, competent to manage their daily lives.
- Children's right to independent use of public space overrides risks from traffic.

These points serve as a basis for discussing how gender and generation intersect in shaping these two models of childhood.

Intersections of gender and generation

Specific to the Nordic societies is the high participation of women in social, economic and political life. A recent worldwide study considered three key issues here: gender equality in enrolment in secondary school (at 95 per cent or more); women's share of paid employment in industry and services (at 50 per cent or more); and women's share of seats in parliament (at 30 per cent or more). Only four countries have achieved all three: Denmark, Finland, Norway and Sweden; and four others come close: Germany, Iceland, the Netherlands and South Africa. The report notes tersely: 'Developed as well as developing countries still have quite a way to go' (United Nations Development Fund for Women 2000: 11).[9]

Women's participation in public life has included, both centrally and as a by-product, challenges to patriarchy, and this is important not only for gender relations but for generational relations (Alanen 1996). The control exercised by male-ordered 'relations of ruling' over the lives of both women and children has been modified by women's increasing power to shape the institutions which organize people's daily lives. These challenges to patriarchy are critical for the development of children's rights. As Therborn's analysis (1993) of the progress of children's rights in European countries indicates, in patriarchal societies women's and children's rights will be subordinated to men's and fathers'. Some versions of Christianity will bolster this control. Thus Catholicism (prevalent in southern European countries) will insist on its primacy above civil law to control people's lives, including family life, whilst weaker versions – such as Lutheranism (in northern European countries) – recognizes the legislative power of the state in family matters. Therborn also discusses a third interrelated strand affecting social developments: the variety of legal bodies and legal thinking across societies. Civil law traditions (which predominate in southern Europe) are more prescriptive and normative, and thereby support the status quo, than common law traditions (prevalent in northern Europe and the UK). These three intersecting strands, patriarchy, religion and law variously affect the advance of both women's and children's rights. Therborn's analysis provides a solid basis for the social reality in Europe: that the Nordic countries have moved furthest on recognizing children's rights, with Anglo-Saxon countries following along, and southern European countries moving more slowly.

The women's movement in the Nordic countries needs emphasis here. It has helped to alter children's lives and bring children and childhood into public consciousness (Therborn 1996). (It is not that women, in fighting for emancipation, have fought for children – for discussion see Chapter 9). There are several ways in which this has happened. Women's work for their own emancipation has included changing 'the family' from a given to a problem; the problem of how responsibility for children's welfare should be divided between 'the family' and the state leads to considerations of what sort of childhoods children should have. The expansion of welfare state services, including daycare, education, health and social services, has meant jobs for women who not only, therefore, participate as workers in public domain, but also contribute to thinking about what services should be provided for children. And in using these services, children's independent participation in social life, including public social life, has increased and made them more visible.

In the UK, the presence of just a few women in high posts in the 1997–2001 parliament can be seen as similarly beginning to shift debates and practices towards the need for and provision of daycare, but also for reconsideration of the balance of paid work and family life for parents – and their children (*Guardian*, Budget Special section, 8 March 2001). But while in Britain patriarchal control continues to subordinate women and children to an important extent, in the Nordic countries women's emancipation has led to weakening of patriarchal power and then to rethinking of both women and children. Children's emergence into public life, as rightful users of services and of public space, has been accompanied by a reconceptualization of children – as citizens with rights. In Finland, specifically, this move has been encouraged by the nation-building enterprises of the twentieth century and especially after World War II. This discussion of intersections of gender and generation is continued in the next, last chapter.

9 | Generation and gender

Generationing processes

If childhood is a social category, participant in structuring the social order, and if childhood is defined in relation to (and contradistinction to) adulthood, then we must study childhood in relational terms, and specifically as determined through processes in generational relations. As I indicated in Chapter 2, I have been influenced by feminism, especially as providing a systematic set of methods for studying a minority social group. Throughout I have given emphasis (see Chapter 3) to the two central questions posed in both history and sociology: How do we account for what we have now? and, How best can we describe what we have now? Critical realism has helped me to understand the relations of structure and agency, the power of established structures and their reproduction and modification through processes of agency–structure interrelations across time. In order to study relational processes, I have taken the principal sites where UK childhoods are lived – the home and the school – and considered both large-scale and long-term, and more local influences on how childhood is understood and actualized and on how children experience and reflect on their daily lives (see Chapters 4 and 5). Much of this book documents processes in thinking from children's lives, working up what they say into an account of their social positioning. Their descriptions and reflections both validate and comment on more ivory tower reflections. Most noticeably, young people give the lie to theories of childhood incompetence and of childhood merely as preparation; young people clearly indicate their moral engagement with issues in relationships both within and across the generations; they put high value on rights, and especially their participation rights, and on interdependence in relationships (see especially Chapters 6 and 7). Another way into understanding relational processes over time, is through comparison, and through consideration of another North European country, I sought to highlight and account for distinctive features of UK childhoods (Chapter 8).

In this chapter, I shall not formally rehearse the substance of the earlier chapters, since I have given summaries and commentaries at the end of each. But I want to take up a number of topics – in the light of those chapters – firstly a topic sketched out in Chapter 3: whether UK children nowadays may be understood as a new generation.

Children as a new generation?

As I briefly outlined in Chapter 3, Mannheim (1952) provides a wide-ranging and comprehensive study of the concept of generation. He writes as a historical sociologist, concerned with cultural history. His problem is to account for cultural change and activity within sociohistorical processes. He argues that though biological generations succeed each other every 30 years or so, social generations are constituted in relation to social change. He discusses three levels of generational identification. People can be seen as similarly *located* where they are exposed to the same phase of important sociohistorical processes, but they vary in their opportunities and in constraints on them as to their thoughts, experiences, and modes of action, and it is social class that differentiates them. A peasant will be differently located from a landowner born at around the same time in the same society. Within generational location, Mannheim sees mechanisms that make for an *actual generation* – where people's experiences, thoughts, attitudes, actions are actuated by specific influences related to their social class position. And finally, a *generational unit* moves beyond this point, for people here form a strong common bond of goals and a programme of action; they realize the potential inherent in their social location, and they 'work up the material of their common experiences' in specific ways (1952: 304).

In line with his own temporal siting in social history, Mannheim conceptualizes youth as the key, formative period of life when people may form an actual generation or generational unit. He makes no reference to gendered social locations; implicitly he is talking about young men. Children had no place in his sociological thought, except as objects of socialization, but we may consider how far his exploration of generation is useful for thinking about childhood. His comprehensive paper provides many suggestive points, of which I focus on four.

First, Mannheim usefully draws attention to variations in how people are exposed to sociohistorical processes, according to their class position. If we accept that children are a distinct social group – or can be understood as a social class in economic terms – exploited by adults at school (Oldman

1994), then it is a short step to thinking of children as being specifically *located*, and having specific experiences of social developments. Examples are many. For instance, it is likely that, if education policy requires 'parental' involvement, children from well-to-do backgrounds will in general gain more than others from this policy. In an age of proliferating technology, those same children will also have better access to computers, both at home and, probably, at school. And, if we live in a risky society where traffic and strangers are ready to pounce and children are confined to their homes, then well-to-do children will again do better – they will have more space at home, with more activities available.

Second, Mannheim's account allows us to consider whether children belong to an *actual generation*. As I have argued in Chapter 7, there is evidence that children do think of themselves as living within a common domain, structured by adult behaviour and interests; they do form solidarity groups – to counter the power of adults at school, and to face up to family change and their own futures. Further, children's accounts indicate that they develop a standpoint on childhood which relates to the specifics of the sociohistorical context within which they are growing up. However it can be strongly argued that children's relative powerlessness within generational relations prohibits their forming a *generational unit*, where people not only form a common bond based on common goals, but can put into practice a programme of activity.

Third, the concept of a formative period for formulating a social con-sciousness throws light on aspects of child–parent relations (see Chapter 4). Parents, who grew up under specific social circumstances, bring to parent–child relations their experience and knowledge. For instance, on the key topic of education, UK parents today remember childhood as a period of freedom and exploration, and school as learning through activity (however dim and distorted their memories). These experiences and memories enter into their relationships with their children. They compensate them for phys-ical restrictions and are angered at today's educational regime, while their children accept the regime as given: that's what school is.

Fourth, Mannheim suggests that where social change is very rapid, the usual latent but continuous adaptation and modification in people's attitudes and actions will give way. Distinctive ways of thinking and action will emerge; the formation of generational units may be facilitated: groups of people with clear visions and programmes. Such rapid social change took place under the UK Conservative governments (1979–97) in the wake of their innovative social policies; these promoted (probably as unintended consequences) changes in adult understandings of childhood. Much more than before, children were to be objects of the education system; their own experiences and interests to be set aside. As child poverty increased so did the demonization of childhood. Significantly for Mannheim's thesis, these understandings and policies were adopted wholesale by the incoming UK Labour government.

These points on Mannheim draw attention to how generational relations structure children's siting as a generation. It is through the processes whereby child–adult relations constitute and reconstitute childhoods that children may be understood as generationally located, or childhood as an actual generation. Children's own agency in constructing childhoods has to be set in the context of adult power to construct them too – the two kinds of agency are in tension.

Childhood in crisis?

Mannheim helps us think about the proposition that childhood is crisis-ridden. As noted in Chapter 1 (pp. 2–4), observers say there has been rapid and menacing change in the conditions in which childhood is lived. I summarize these proposed changes as context for the thesis that children nowadays constitute a new generation.

Probably the overriding perceived large-scale development in recent years is people's understanding that they live in a 'risk society' (Beck 1992), where risk is omnipresent and out of their control (a polluted environment, nuclear proliferation, multinational interests, capitalism itself). Locally this means people perceive the outside world as dangerous, parents restrict children more than they themselves remember being (Chapter 4). Though there are no data from children from earlier generations on this, and though parents' memories may be faulty, it does seem that a dramatic change has taken place. Within the risk society, the notion of the individualization of people's careers (away from predetermined careers based on parental socio-economic position) leads to the notion of individual responsibility for success. Certainly the current education system promotes this view; parents in the Risk Study agonized over choice of school to maximize their children's academic chances, and the young people accepted their individual respons-ibility for their futures (Chapter 5).

The huge increase in child poverty in the UK during the Conservative years (1979–97) from about 10 per cent to about 30 per cent means that social class, defined according to income, continues to affect children's life-chances, more seriously than in more equal European societies. The current Labour government claims to have reduced the numbers from four to three million during its first term (1997–2001) and plans further reductions, but meanwhile children living in poverty are more likely than others to die in early childhood, eat poorer food, be excluded from school, leave school without qualifications, engage in crime, suffer mental disorder. Such inequalities by income mean that for every topic some children will be systematically disadvantaged (Lansdown 1995).

There is also evidence suggesting rapid processes of change in the gendering of child–parent relations. Whilst Mum may always have been the linchpin of households (?), the feminization of families (Jensen 1994) seems to have proceeded apace (Burns 1995); increasing proportions of children grow up with women rather than with women and men, and some people are therefore concerned about the health of boys (e.g. O'Donnell and Sharpe 2000). Mothers' triple responsibilities – for breadwinning, for family welfare, and for involvement with the school – may affect their relations with both their daughters and their sons. Young people reported far more conversations with mothers than with fathers (see also Langford *et al.* 2001; Ribbens McCarthy 2001) and though most expressed the normative view that mothers' main job was caring for the family, many were relating in practice to mothers who did paid work; child–parent relations could be adversely affected by homework demands.

And finally there have been major rapid changes in the media technologies available to children. As David Buckingham describes, the prophets of doom vie with the optimists (2000: *passim* and summarized in Chapter 10). The doom-merchants foresee the death of childhood as children are exposed to 'adult entertainment' and are stressed beyond their years; the optimists see children as liberated from adult-controlled childhoods through their access to knowledge, entertainment and networks of children. Buckingham argues that the evidence for a full-blown acceptance of either thesis is poor, and that the claimants exaggerate their theses (for discussion, see also Kline 2001). But he does see children and childhood being pulled simultaneously in two directions: children are being empowered through technology, but they are also increasingly institutionalized. Further, the increasing commercialization and privatization of the media again increases inequalities since children vary in their access both to the various forms of the new media, and to other sources of amusement and learning – such as books and conversation. Both material and social capital affect what children can gain from new and old sources.

Arguably, children nowadays are uniquely *located* in relation to intersections of these developments. They probably are located as a new generation in the risk society. Compared to 30 years ago, childhoods are more sharply polarized by parental income. Girls and boys are growing up alongside new ways of living as a woman and as a man, and these changes may influence their beliefs and actions both now and later. The new media are commonplace to them, probably not central to their lives (in most cases), but providing both opportunities and dangers (Valentine *et al.* 2000; Hutchby and Moran-Ellis 2001).

Perhaps too children form an *actual generation*, since, clearly, they engage with the social structures they identify around them, making the best of good things available to them and coping with the worst. But while they deal with the new, their main concerns are very traditional; most important to them are that they have good relationships with at least one parent and with people at school. Young people in other studies also rate good personal relationships highly (see Chapter 4: 62).

On the other hand, as indicated especially in Chapters 5, 6 and 7, young people's accounts suggest cause for concern at present. They found that adults both defined them as morally incompetent and demanded that they be competent (and I saw gaps between their ascribed incompetence and their moral competence in practice).[1] They argued for their rights to the three Ps: protection, provision and participation, and identified marked adult failings as to participation, with schools especially at fault. Unlike some commentators, these young people did not suggest they were being rushed into adulthood; indeed most enjoyed childhood as a privileged period of life. However, they identified very clear boundaries round childhood and adulthood, with adults rightly having authority over children; they experienced the outside world as dangerous and accepted adult protection, but this led to constant negotiations about permission to go out, and in some cases to conflict. Essentially, these points concern children's moral status in the processes of child–adult interactions.

Promoting children's rights

Children's rights are increasingly a topic for discussion, and the literature increases by the day.[2] My main contribution here has been in arguing for including childhood as a constituent and active component of the social order. I follow Knutsson (1997) in suggesting that one may raise the status of childhood through arguing for and demonstrating children's social responsibilities; improved status may lead to respect for their rights.

Respect for children's rights is certainly lacking, specifically in the UK (Children's Rights Development Unit 1994). Yet, as Franklin (1995) points out, neither of the main opposing arguments stands up well. The first accusation, that children lack competence, falls against the evidence that, whilst children may have less experience than adults, and may in some respects and on some occasions be learning their way, they seriously engage with moral issues and contribute to constructing the social order, from the earliest days (e.g. Alderson 2000a). It seems that those who work for children must keep on describing and analysing this engagement, in order to help shift people away from denigrating children's moral abilities, and towards recognizing their ability – as well as desire – to participate in decision-making. The second argument, that children may make mistakes, applies to adults too, and anyway, you cannot learn without practice. An important practical move here would be to lower the voting age, for instance to 16 (Lindley 1989; Scarre 1989b; Freeman 2000); this would at least mean that the voices of some of those still in school could be heard in political arenas.

It is clear that children's views should form part of policy-related discussions on current topics. Critical at present is the division of people's time between work, 'the family' and leisure pursuits. Many children told me they valued time spent with parents (not a topic on policy agendas). As has recently been suggested by some observers (including Labour MPs), the nine to five day in paid work is not a necessary norm to which all should conform; flexibility and choice could surely be achieved for people of all ages. Childcare – for the youngest children – would be considerably less of a problem if parents had such choices.[3] Young people's work towards getting an education does not need to be all day and every day in an institution.

The UK is slowly moving towards better paid leave for parents after a child is born, but much more needs to be done both here and even in the Nordic countries to allow people, including children, more freedom to choose how and where to spend time.[4] (The double shift of Nordic women continues – full-time work and childcare/domestic responsibility at home.) We could allow teenagers and 65-year-olds to go to work, and release more of the time of parents. Some tentative steps are being taken on letting teenagers mix school and paid work, and on retaining older workers up to, for instance, 72 years (*Independent*, 25 March 2001).

As to 'the school', young people's wishes and perspectives are desperately needed to crack the present impasse. For whilst commentators argue that we need a flexible, creative, problem-solving workforce, educationalists in England and Wales increasingly institutionalize childhood, and prioritize adult agendas and student conformity. Furthermore current policies that try to make all children conform to school as so organized are clearly counterproductive, as well as expensive. Some commentators suggest, however, that the current school will have to give way to the technological revolution, and that students as learners and choosers, creating their own programme of study and activity, may emerge. Bentley (1998), for instance, argues for the school as a hub, to be used by people of all ages, where students each have a tutor who helps them map out a programme of work, which they then implement using locally available resources (libraries, sport facilities, the internet, community centres, universities). Such a vision still assumes that young people want to learn, but that seems a sounder basis for an educational vision (since young children at least seem passionately keen to learn) than the notion that they will all conform to fixed adult agendas. A 2001 poll of children's views indicated that they value education, and want schools with good physical conditions, democratic ethos and respect for children as learners.[5]

Critical to developing a society where people can exercise choice is their ownership of public space. Blaming parents for restricting children's mobility or the media for whipping up stranger-danger scares will not solve the problem. What is required is the political will to open up space to people, and that must include children's participation in planning for children's mobility, literally on the ground; plenty of schemes already exist, but are insufficiently implemented: home zones, reductions in traffic, speed restrictions, safe routes to schools. Changing the material and social character of public space are essential for changing ideas about who has the right to use it. It is only when conditions are physically safe and welcoming that people in general will spend time out and about, and that children too will be accepted as rightful users of public space.

More generally, I refer to the important paper by Gerison Lansdown (1995), who reviewed the lessons she and colleagues learned from their work towards a report on the state of children's rights in the UK (Lansdown and Newell 1994). She makes four main points. The principal message from young people was that they felt powerless, not listened to, not respected. Discrimination against children was rife in all areas of UK society and institutions. Poverty and the consequences for children's lives now and for the future was a dominant theme emerging from the work. Inadequate support for parents in caring for children and promoting their rights was a serious impediment to their contribution.[6] The UK's second Report (1999) to the UN Committee on the CRC indicates some progress since then towards appointing Commissioners for Children in Scotland, Northern Ireland and Wales. Judging by the Report, resistance seems strongest in English government circles, where the child as problem (victim or threat) holds sway. The Report ignores the Committee's advice to respect children's participation rights. However, there are encouraging initiatives: voluntary childcare organizations have forefronted children's rights; membership of the European Union has led to challenges to UK policies and practices (for instance on hitting children). A new EU Charter of Fundamental Rights (signed December 2000) summarizes children's rights to protection, care and participation, with the child's best interests a primary consideration (Article 24).

As suggested in Chapter 8, patriarchal structures are the principal barriers to recognition of children's rights. And, as *The Human Rights of Women and Children* (UNICEF 1998) points out, on some issues these two subordinated groups face similar problems and 'can teach each other how to tackle them'; in particular the report draws attention to the worldwide problem of ensuring that women and children 'can overcome those conservative appeals to culture, tradition, religion and customs' and decide for themselves whether and to what extent they wish to live their lives in accordance with them (UNICEF 1998: 12). Further, the report argues, some issues raise dilemmas which can be addressed only through consideration of the rights of both women and children; for instance children's rights to breastfeeding and mothers' right to go out to work; the rights of children born from rape to know their parents and mothers' rights to integrity; girls' rights to education and women's rights not to suffer a double workload. In such cases careful interpretation of the two relevant conventions can avoid conflict and respect the rights of each (see also Freeman 2000).

Towards a sociology for childhood

In Chapter 2, I paid tribute to the work of feminists, notably Margaret Stacey and Dorothy Smith, who argued that study of women's lives must include study of intersections with children's lives or, more grandly and radically, that study of the division of labour must take account of children's contributions. Here I take up these themes as central towards constructing a sociology for childhood.

Is feminism interested in childhood?

The first issue is whether we can directly derive useful ideas from feminism when trying to theorize childhood. This leads on to some questions: whether feminist thinkers have interested themselves first in children as persons and second in childhood as a constituent category in the social order. Early reviews of the literature (Ramazanoglu 1989; Leonard 1990) indicate an adult-only focus in feminism, with a few notable exceptions where age as well as gender feature.[7] More recent feminist accounts from the English-speaking world – written after 15 years of sociological development on childhood – indicate that they are not influenced by such work.[8] Generally feminists do not discuss childhood, but emphasize mothers' childcare work; women may construe children as valuable, but they also constitute a job.[9] Thus for Lynne Segal (1995), who reviews the stages of feminist work, the central issue is the status of women and how this can be improved; adult gender relations are the topic. Feminist analyses of 'the family' focus almost exclusively on adult gender relations, adult paid work and childcare responsibilities. Thus Valerie Bryson (1999: Ch. 6) argues for 'a better balance for all' but children figure in her discussion only as depersonalized objects of childcare (see also Carol Lee Bacchi 1999). Feminist studies of educational issues identify gender as the fundamental underlying concept through which experience, process and outcome may be understood (see papers in Holland et al. 1995; David et al. 1997).

Children and childhood as topics of interest for feminists did emerge in the 1980s, in discussions of patriarchal power over both women and children within 'the home' (Delphy 1984). More recently Lynne Segal (1999: 206–11) argues that the abuse of women and children within the nuclear family is masked and denied through the Labour Party's support for 'the family', with the complementary rhetoric, implied by Labour and overt in the media, that non-nuclear families – 'fatherless' children, 'divorced families' and 'lone parent families' – constitute social problems and inadequate 'parenting'. But childhood as a constituent part of the social order, generational issues and children as people with interests, rights and contributions are not, in general, a focus for feminism (see the initial discussion on feminist theory in Chapter 2). In seeking an explanation for feminists' neglect of theoretical initiatives on childhood, Leena Alanen (1992: 32–3) argues that they (like mainstream sociologists) have uncritically accepted developmental models of children's 'needs', so if psychologists said children 'need' maternal care then feminist thinkers had to define children as 'adversaries' of women. Perhaps we should take account too of differing ideologies underpinning family policies. In North America, Australasia and the UK, where the state provides only for extreme 'welfare cases', women's battle to escape the demands of social motherhood, and win employment and career and political engagement, is a battle to free themselves from the social assignment to mothers of childcare responsibilities. Feminists think they must push children aside in the interests of advancing women's rights. In mainland Europe, by contrast, policy measures to support early childcare at home, to provide daycare services after the first year or so, and to encourage fathers to share in domestic childcare allow feminists to focus (relatively) untrammelled on gender issues in adult relations in both the 'public' and 'private' spheres: the continuing gendered inequalities in pay and careers, in political life, and in the domestic division of childcare. Since the state takes responsibility for providing daycare services, parents are relieved of that responsibility during the day. The interests, including the rights, of children are a separate agenda, dealt with by a different constituency, and by other policies.

In both sorts of society, the division of responsibility for children seems to distract feminists' (and men's) attention from children as persons and from childhood as social status.[10] Children and childhood remain a childcare and daycare issue. In the UK, post-war debates on whether maternal care or others' care is best for young children raged for over 30 years (see e.g. Leach 1979) but have died down somewhat since the early 80s, largely because policies that impoverished families have resulted in the dire necessity for mothers to bring income into their families (Oppenheim and Lister 1996) and so demoted the relatively minor matter of the quality of children's experience during the day.[11] By contrast, in mainland Europe it has become an accepted fact of life that children will spend most of their days, from their second year, in daycare. This social acceptance of the institutionalization of young children has reduced interest in alternatives, but has allowed service-providers to develop democratic practices.[12] Implementing democratic principles in daycare centres has always been easier than in schools, since policymakers are less prescriptive for the youngest children. But the societal assumption is that parents will re-enter the labour force after a year or so's leave (Moss 1997); and, arguably, these childhoods are subordinated to adulthood, feminist goals and/or national economic prosperity.

Feminism and childhood studies

At this point, however, I pay belated tribute to a relatively minor stream in feminist thought; work which has, since the early 1980s, outlined rationales for taking account of children and childhood. It is within philosophical studies of feminism that scholars have somewhat widened their vision to include children, notably by considering children as people whose rights should be respected. Janet Radcliffe Richards (1980: 310–17) argues that children should not be seen (as in some feminist writing) as commodities whose care falls on women but whose value is to the society; children should be seen as having rights – and therefore the state should ensure 'that their needs are met', through providing services and benefits which target children (income support, daycare, health, education). Jean Bethke Elshtain (1981: 348) briefly includes children in her discussion of citizenship and participation towards reforms of the social order. Alison Jaggar, discussing socialist feminism, notes its assumptions that people, from birth onwards, engage in self-creation, and that early childhood is a formative time of life. On grounds of respect for children as persons, and also, pragmatically, because those persons will be the adults of the future, she argues:

> Taken together, these views suggest that children must be fully active participants in making the decisions that affect them most directly and so participate in controlling their own lives . . . Children are smaller and weaker than adults; they are less skilled and have less information. Like adults, however, they create their own nature through their own forms of daily praxis. Both the dignity of children now and a concern for the future society they will construct require that revolutionaries take seriously the notion of extending democracy to children. Of course they should include children in those reflections.
>
> (Jaggar 1983: 343)

Barrie Thorne (1987) gives perhaps the fullest consideration in the 1980s of the need to include children and childhood within feminist thought. She argues for consideration of the complex intertwining of age and gender categories, for deconstruction of ideologies of childhood and attention to varieties of childhood experience, and for full exploration of children as social agents. With remarkable prescience, she argues that children must be regarded as agents negotiating with institutional structures, across private and public domains.

These points were taken up by Leena Alanen in her analysis of 'the child question in feminism'(1992: 26). Her study also analyses ways in which the methods of feminism (critique, deconstruction, conceptual development, standpoint) can be applied in childhood studies. And her empirical study of children's daily lives in lone mother households draws attention to their constructive agency in shaping their experience in intersection and negotiation with their mothers.

These provocative analyses provide the basis for the discussion in the rest of this chapter. Like these pioneers, I would argue that feminists must take part in the retheorizing of childhood in relation to adulthood, and thus give serious attention to the social status, social positioning and contributions of the various social groups that construct the social order. Otherwise they cannot move towards a comprehensive account of gender and generation as implicated in structuring the social order. Feminists have typically seen children as a cause of their own oppression. But what is needed is thinking towards social understandings whose structures do not deprive some people of freedom in order to give it to others (Lansdown 1995). Such thinking involves recognition that children are people (rather than objects of concern) with rights; that children themselves have views on how childhood should be lived; that children contribute to the division of labour both within 'families' and in the wider social order; and that child–parent relations have varying characteristics and meanings across the lifespan.[13]

During the course of this book, I have proceeded through a set of stages, as developed in feminist thought. These stages include first critiquing the status quo; then considering how to deconstruct it, through developing an analysis of a key concept – generational relations; and finally working towards a child standpoint. Thus the early parts of the book (especially Chapter 2) outlined the critiques that have been mounted of traditional sociological understandings of childhood, and discussed differences between recent psychological and sociological concerns about childhood. The deconstruction of traditional, badly fitting concepts of childhood involves developing a concept (analagous to gender in feminism) – generation – as a means of providing a better set of understandings of childhood. Discussion of generational relations proceeds through the book, with emphasis on the continued impact of the past on the present. The four central chapters give considerable space to children's own experiences and understandings, and move towards outlining a child standpoint. Chapter 8 uses comparison across countries to highlight some key factors structuring the sociopolitical status quo of UK childhoods.

In the task of upgrading childhood, adult recognition of the agency of children is central. Such recognition has been long in coming, but there is now a proliferation of studies which identify and discuss agency; indeed young people's agency has enabled researchers to do this work easily. Linked to this is the overdue discovery that whilst young people may never have heard of the UN Convention on the Rights of the Child, they talk from their earliest years in rights terms – of protection, provision and participation, of fairness, justice, respect for others, and interdependence. The concept of children as moral agents means we have to recognize childhood as a permanent social category, childhood contributions to the division of labour and childhood as standing in a specific relation to other social categories, which may be represented through a child standpoint.

As I noted in Chapter 2, women have developed three linked themes that seem especially useful to explore: the division of labour, the intermediate domain, and standpoint theory. Through considering children's and childhood's contributions to the construction of the social order, in relation to adult contributions, I am trying to develop ways of bringing feminism and childhood studies together, and so to provide a more adequate account of processes in the structuring of the social order.

Children in the division of labour
I see two strands here: children as workers at school, and children engaged in people work at home and school. On the basis of analysis of large-scale trends in industrialized countries, Qvortrup (1985, 1995, 2001) argues that children's participation in the labour force is now to be understood through their activity as learners, defined as work. His historical analysis describes the removal of children from the paid workforce, and argues for their inclusion in the division of labour through their participation in learning, most clearly seen in their schoolwork.

Defining some of children's activities as work is less a matter of stretching the concept of work to include children's activities within established notions of the public and the private; it is more a matter of critiquing the public–private divide. Childhood has been constituted as a site of education to be carried out in homes and schools, with mothers working in both, for their children and for the education system, and children as agents also working on self-capitalization in both; this means that notions of public and private give way to a vision of activity, taking place in distinctive spaces and times, but as an integrated composite programme of activity towards the goal of the educated person. (This is not to say that young people themselves do not resist this integration; in my personal and research experience, they do; they say home and school differ; the home is freer and should be so; they resist mother and teacher incursions into their 'free time' at home; see Chapter 5.) The point I am making here is that concepts of the proper activities of childhood, at this point in the UK's history of educational policy, serve to blur demarcations between 'public' and 'private'. Indeed, I think one can go further, and question the notion that the preschool and school (at least for the early years) are firmly sited within a 'public' domain. The very notion of the crucial importance of mothers' contribution to their children's education serves to site the school in an intermediate domain, where staff negotiate with mothers, and take account of children's own knowledge and interests where their models of childhood permit.

The argument that children's activity at school is work can be supported by theoretical analysis of how social groups contribute to the division of labour in society. Children can be understood as acquiring, through inter-action with teachers, the skills and knowledge required for their effective participation in social life and in paid work. David Oldman (1994) defines children's school activity as self-capitalization, but thinks it is devalued as part of the process of adult exploitation of children's work at school. It is noteworthy that some children have absorbed the view that what they do at school is not work (see Chapter 5) – a tribute to the power of Durkheim's assumption that schoolchildren are in a preparatory stage of life, being made fit, through socialization, to join (adult) society (1961: 17–19). Children's agency in their own learning is of fundamental, and neglected, importance in the UK; for as Paolo Freire proposes (1996: *passim*, and especially Ch. 3), the essential function of schools is for staff to work with children towards children's engagement with their sociohistorical position and towards their active participation in the creation of their culture.[14]

The second strand in children's contribution to the division of labour links understandings of children as agents with feminist contentions that much of women's work, paid or unpaid, is 'people work' (see p. 11). Academic discourses in psychology and sociology (as discussed in Chapter 6) have drawn attention to children's active participation, from their early months, in the construction of knowledge and of the social order at home and in pre-school. Research in the natural setting of the home has shown that children can be understood as participants in the construction of know-ledge. They participate with parents and sibs in the construction and recon-struction of the social order of the home through identifying and refining issues of justice, fair distribution, kindness and recognition of others' points of view. They act as reasonable people. They may do practical, caring people work; for instance in Burke and Montgomery's study (2001) 80 per cent of children participated in caring for their disabled sib. In pre-schools, those adults who take children seriously, again as participants in demo-cratic orders, find that children contribute enthusiastically and responsibly both in considering agendas for the centre's work and in constructing friend-ships (Corsaro 1996; Malaguzzi 1998; Clark and Moss 2001).

My own research work has demonstrated that children contribute in other ways to the household division of labour and to constructing the social order of the home. They do this through taking on self-care activities, whereby they establish themselves as competent members of the family, and also free up mothers' time. They also contribute to the family work order by carrying out housework (cf. Zelizer 1985: 209). Solberg (1990) points to both gender and generation as factors (Norwegian data); women do most housework, then girls, then boys, and men least. In ways that are more difficult to quantify, I argue that children contribute through making, maintaining and improving relationships with others at home, and in many cases with relatives who live elsewhere – such as fathers and grandparents (see also Brannen *et al.* 2000). Young people's accounts show that they not only empathize with those they live with, but take responsibility for their welfare – 'sentient activity' in Jennifer Mason's (1996) terms. Through discussions and storytelling they learn about their parents' childhoods and later histories, and how these histories form part of parents' thinking about their children's lives now and their futures; in some cases (for instance, Alan, p. 50) children express clear feelings of responsibility for carrying forward their parents' hopes.

Some of this work takes the form of support, much of it at home in alliance with mothers (see Chapter 4). Thus children and mothers work through issues in their respective lives, clear examples being discussions about changes in who lives where – when fathers move out, stepfathers and babies move in. This is mutually confiding work, mainly between children and their mothers (less commonly their fathers). Where family members are facing difficulties, such as illness (as Sandra described on p. 90), disability (Burke and Montgomery 2001), migration (Candappa 2000a), divorce (Smart and Neale 2000a), young people's accounts indicate clearly that they both give and receive help. Furthermore, in their interrelations with each other young people show how they provide support, make common cause, make sense of experiences and construct solidarity as a minority social group. At home the children may act together in tension, conflict or negotiation with parents, to put the child viewpoint, to support and comfort each other. At school, where power relations between adults and children are powerfully and sometimes rigidly enforced, young people's accounts indicate the central importance of solidarity with the child group.

Thus mainstream historical analysis combined with feminist analysis provides us with the means to include children in the division of labour, through their school work and through their relationships with important adults at school and at home. The structuring of women's daily lives through ideologies and policies ensures that, in the UK, it will be women with whom children mainly interact, learn, negotiate and construct relationships.

The intermediate domain
At suggested above, we must critique the notion of the social order as composed of public and private domains, yet more forcefully, once we think of children as participants in constructing the social order. We have

become accustomed to the idea that women's work crosses the 'public' and the 'private', managing their bodily experience in both (Martin 1989) and working for their children in transactions and interactions with health staff (Stacey and Davies 1983) and school staff (Smith 1988; Mayall 1994). Women transfer caring skills acquired in their work at home to nursing and teaching jobs (Graham 1983). In recent years, there are increasing policy demands that mothers work at home on their children towards realization of school agendas (see Chapter 5). Thus consideration of women's activities suggests that the notion of the 'public' and 'private' makes little sense and then only if one looks at traditional (and stereotypical) men's lives.

The concept of the intermediate domain is important here (Stacey and Davies 1983; and see Chapter 2, this volume, p. 11). Whilst human service activities – or people work – take place in both the 'public' and the 'private' domains (as demarcated in classical sociology texts), it is useful to conceptualize a space between the two where paid and unpaid people, mostly women, work together in the interests of better services. At issue, crucially, is the status of women's knowledge, and key sites are health and education services, where mothers and staff negotiate the status of their knowledge and experience. The intermediate domain provides a conceptual space for understanding the complexities of relations between the public and the private in highly developed welfare states – it provides a means of analysing intersections of state and family; it provides a tool for dissolving the notion of two opposed domains, and of studying how far 'lay' and 'professional' knowledge, goals and practices affect each other.

I have suggested that children too act in an intermediate domain, where they too propose their knowledge, experience, goals and practices as relevant to planning and provision by those who provide services 'for' them. Crucial here is the power of adults to determine how far children have agency.[15] Children's participation rights have varying status across social welfare, health and education services. As Gerison Lansdown (1995) notes, the Children Act 1989 requires providers of social services to take account of children's views, but the Act applies to only a small minority of children, and evidence indicates that so far compliance with this requirement is patchy. In the health and education sectors there is no such requirement, and to date UK governments have been complacent about their failure to comply with the CRC.[16] At one extreme, agencies may implement democratic principles by building children's participation into the ethos, guidelines, staff training and practices of the service; at the other, they may deliberately exclude children's participation as irrelevant to the adult-devised purposes of the service. Nursery schools in the UK have traditionally operated on democratic principles (Penn 2000). Significantly however, in the increasingly instrumental education policy climate, they are steadily being closed as uneconomic and children are being diverted to nursery classes in schools, where the regime is more adult-led, more oriented to preparation for school.

I argued in Chapter 5 that school agendas, controlled by teachers under national education policies, prioritize the cognitive over the bodily and emotional in schools, and that children have little power to maintain the control over pacing their day that they have at home. Children's resistance to adult demands and the adult-ordered day may be limited to small adjustments and 'time-shifting' devices (Christensen and James 2001) to alleviate tedium and strain. In terms of the formal curriculum, the question whether respect for children's own knowledge is commonplace in school remains to be fully explored. My own research experiences in primary schools forcibly indicate that adult agendas are pre-eminent. Whilst children's knowledge, experience and skill may generally have low status at school, one would think that they would be understood as relevant when topics in personal and social education, including citizenship, are under consideration. Yet teachers may find it hard to do this. Priscilla Alderson (2000c) found both good and bad practice; some teachers wished to practise as well as preach rights, but were hampered by senior staff and the established social order of the school; others apparently saw no conflict between their preaching and rights-denying practice.

Young people's participation in the intermediate domain is hard to identify, since it is an unfamiliar idea. Young people are not generally understood as having relevant knowledge to contribute to modifying their own and others' lives. But young people act as mediators between home and school, in connection with parental involvement and homework (p. 81; Edwards and Alldred 2000), and in considering their futures (for example, Asian girls, p. 130); together with their mothers, they contribute to improving the quality of their own daily experience, across home and school (Stuart, p. 83). Where, for various reasons, young people take on work generally regarded as inappropriate for childhood, they may negotiate directly with agencies for themselves or for others (Barry 2001); for instance 'young carers', who look after disabled sibs and parents, may have to negotiate the status of their knowledge and perceived needs with welfare agencies in order to get help (Dearden *et al.* 1994; Aldridge and Becker 1995). UK-born children of immigrants may act as interpreters and advocates for themselves and their parents. Other key groups of young people are those who are disabled (Appleton 1995; Watson 2000), and 'in care' (Wilson 1995). At issue is their ability to make their knowledge known and respected. The power of service-providers to control knowledge and services is crucial when young people ask for services, for they have even less power than adult help-seekers to control what happens next; some young people are unwilling to discuss problematic issues with welfare agencies, since to do so is to hand over the knowledge to those with power to control it (Williamson and Butler 1995; see also Davies and Cloke

1995; Sandbaek 1999). As Mano Candappa (2000b) points out, in her study of refugee children, the school is the agency to which they all (?) go, and it is therefore the best placed to help them: by listening to their concerns, and by providing a learning environment which helps them settle in, feel normal again and learn English. She too found examples of both good and of bad practice in schools.

In sum, the notion of an intermediate domain is useful for considering young people's negotiation of knowledge and perceived needs with agencies; it provides a theoretical umbrella for the increasing number of studies which document young people's participation in negotiating with agencies. Young people's participation in the division of labour must be seen to include their intermediate domain work.

Standpoint
On standpoint theory:

> it is not the experiences or the speech that provides the grounds for feminist claims; it is rather the subsequently articulated observations of and theory about the rest of nature and social relations – observations and theory that start out from, that look at the world from the perspective of, women's lives.
>
> (Harding 1991: 124)

As Sandra Harding puts it, women as a minority group constitute 'valuable strangers' (1991: 124). Women's accounts point to disjunctions, flaws, injustices and gaps in conceptual schemes and dominant institutions, whereas men's accounts fit too closely with them. So too with children in relation to adults. The importance of the standpoint of minority groups is in giving a better account of how society works, than is given by the ruling classes, since it comes closer to representing the interests of society as a whole (Jaggar 1983: 370). So we can assert that child standpoints are essential to giving a good account, and are to be considered in relation to adult standpoints.

Crucially, intersections of generation and gender must be studied. Extending Jaggar's argument (1983: 385), I add to her point (in italics): 'the knowledge generated is useful if it contributes to a practical reconstruction of the world – in which women's interests are not subordinated to those of men' *and in which children's interests are not subordinated to adults'*.

In Chapter 6 I focused on the moral status of childhood, and on the mixed messages young people receive about it; on the one hand they are routinely denigrated as morally incompetent, but on the other hand they are, equally routinely, expected to behave well. And furthermore, their accounts demonstrate their moral agency beyond what adults generally expect of them; in relationships with other children and with adults they demonstrate that they have well established moral abilities, recognition of others' points of view, empathy and willingness to give time to others' problems. Generally they do not give themselves credit for their moral competence, and in this they have accepted their lowly social status. In Chapter 7, I discussed what kind of whole the accounts of young people add up to; my description focused on commonality in their accounts, and on their analysis of childhood. My own description of what they say gives a particular shape to it; it relies on my own experience over the years of young people talking and on my analysis of their social positioning. In shaping their accounts, I am trying to follow the precepts of feminists in their discussions of standpoint (Smith 1988; Harding 1991; Alanen 1992; Maynard 1998). As yet, there has been very little development of the notion of standpoint in childhood studies. So what I have argued here is tentative, and should be subject to findings from other studies as they emerge.

Once we accept childhood as a permanent social category, then the notion of child standpoint is important for proper understanding of the social order. This is not to argue for one standpoint; it is to accept, as feminisms have, that standpoint varies according to sociopolitical positioning, and so that children have in common, broadly, a position structured by the specific, local, organization of social relations.[17] So theoretically we will have to consider how children's standpoints demand shifts in sociological understandings. Notably, in the light of child agency we must rethink the notion of childhood as preparation. Given childhood participation in the division of labour we must rethink the sociology of the family and develop our understandings of work as a constituent part of childhood. We shall have to revisit the concept of the intermediate domain to consider childhood's contributions. As this book has argued throughout, we shall have to enlarge the categories with which we analyse the social order to include generation, and analysts of gender will have to consider intersections with generation.

In terms of policy development, we need, of course, more data from children. The data from my studies – with only a few children – provide just a glimpse of how the social world children live in looks from their point of view. Their view is both more pragmatic – acceptance of lowly, apprenticeship status – and more critical than that of some adult observers and analysers. In practical, policy terms, this double vision requires reconsideration of adult–child relations and institutional structures. To develop a child standpoint is to make one kind of move towards upgrading childhood; it is to propose that children's own take on their social positioning is worthy of attention and consideration. It is 'an equality project' (Alanen 1992: 108). For instance, if children feel subordinated (however rightly) to adults, then we adults must reconsider the legitimacy for this imposition of subordination. If young people think of childhood, also, as a period of privilege, and if we adults agree it should be so, then we must consider measures to decrease social inequalities between childhoods, to alleviate poverty, to provide health and education and social services, and to make public space safe for everyone. If being a child means not receiving respect for one's views, we should consider whether the boundaries between adulthood and childhood are too strong – the cases of children in the education system and of 'young carers' acutely raise this issue. What 'my' London children say about the merits of childhood draws attention to the social conditions of children who are less fortunate, and what they say about their experience of the neglect of their rights is a necessary corrective and one which only they can supply; their accounts should feed into measures towards respect for their rights.

Working for childhood

The aim of the sociological enterprise in respect of children and childhood is to provide a reasoned account of how children can be understood as contributors – as moral agents, as workers – and beyond that point, how childhood can be understood as contributory to the social order. Like feminism for women, the sociology of childhood is working for children. This does not mean that the knowledge generated is necessarily available to all children – probably most children, like most women, will not read the tomes emerging in the respective fields. But the simple, central points – that children are moral agents, that they think they should, and do participate in constructing the social order – these emerge in what they say and can be worked up into a standpoint, through setting them within social analysis.

The principal aim of developing sociological thinking about childhood is to contribute to raising the status of childhood; it aims to be sociology for childhood. In this case, I have drawn on the insights of historical sociology, in siting explanations for the present condition of childhood in the sedimented structures of the past, still influential in the present. And I have emphasized a relational sociology, where one is concerned with processes through which, following critical realism, structures are reproduced or modified. By considering childhood as a relational concept, we can contribute towards a better understanding of the social order. This book is a contribution aimed at improving childhood. It is for childhood, in favour of higher status for childhood, and in complement for better distribution of resources to childhood.

| Notes

Chapter 1 Introduction

1 Mills gives a very useful account of 'Intellectual Craftsmanship' in an appendix to *The Sociological Imagination*, but, with hindsight, he reveals the (inevitable) limitations of his own imaginative vision, over a lifetime's work. His vision did not stretch to take full account of women, and children are nowhere.

2 During the years 1988–98 I applied to the Economic and Social Research Council for funds to explore childhood; in all I wrote 18 proposals. Of these, three theoretical and policy-oriented studies were funded; also a seminar series (with Alan Prout), which was valuable as a forum for developing ideas; and a Research Fellowship, which is allowing me time to write this book (5 of 18 or 28 per cent). I also failed to get funds from other agencies, notably on children's management of chronic conditions (asthma, diabetes) across the home and school.

3 For notes on research work with children, see Appendix (p. 190).

Chapter 2 Studying childhood

1 For use of the terms 'childcare' and 'daycare' see the Appendix (p. 191).

2 The concept of 'people work' was developed by Goffman in his study of asylums, where he details how staff operationalize total institutions: 'they are the forcing house for changing persons; each is a natural experiment on what can be done to the self' (1968: 22).

3 A referee on one of my unsuccessful research proposals observed that no useful data could be collected from people as young as 12 years old.

4 Details about the four studies (samples, methods) are given in the Appendix.

5 For discussions of mother-teacher relations carried out by Dorothy Smith's colleagues, see Griffith 1995 and Manicom 1995.

6 For a range of perspectives on this topic, see: Harré 1986; Ingleby 1986; Morss 1990; Prout and James 1990; Urwin and Sharland 1992; Burman 1994; Hendrick 1994: Chapter 5; Jenks 1996: 36–43.

7 Important work on this topic includes: Hart 1997; Cockburn 1998; Johnson *et al.* 1998; Alderson 2000a, 2000b; and Smith *et al.* 2000.

8 Commentators have pointed out drawbacks to Smith's arguments (e.g. Layder 1994: 158–64). By insisting on the micro, she cuts out possibilities for collecting other kinds of data – such as surveys and controlled trials, which may improve understanding of women's social status (Maynard 1998; Oakley 2000). She tends to assume, rather than to arrive at through analysis, her 'relations of ruling', so her claims that she works upwards from women's experience mask this assumed agenda. Her work is also a bit static, in that it gives little space to process and interaction.

Chapter 3 Studying relational processes

1 I give *The German Ideology* quotation with reference to the 1970 edition. Bhaskar (1979) quotes an earlier edition (1965: 65) in his Chapter 2, Note 34.

2 As outlined in Chapter 1, some onlookers regard present-day western childhoods as distinctive, and some think childhood is in crisis.

3 My automatic spell-checker still does not recognize the term gendering. More forgivably, it has not met the term generationing.

4 Generationed is another word not known to the spell-checker.

5 Spell-checker again having problems – with operationalize.

6 Usage of the term 'child' is discussed in the Appendix (p. 191).

Chapter 4 Relations with parents

1 See Appendix (p. 191) for a note on usage of the term 'child'.

2 The points made in this section come from interviews with children aged 5–13: in the Greenstreet Study (5/6 and 9/10), the Risk Study (9/10 and 12/13) and the Childhood Study (9/10 and 12/13).

3 In my studies, it was generally the case that parents' separation took place up to the end of their children's primary school years. So it was younger rather than older children who were dealing with the immediate changes. The older ones had more experience of fathers' neglect as the years of separation wore on.

4 These studies took place during and in the aftermath of 18 years of Conservative rule, during which poverty levels rose markedly. Child poverty rose from about 10 to about 30 per cent (Rahman 2000; Hood 2001).

5 This notion of parental responsibility for shaping childhood and for what the child will become runs very deep in western thought. By contrast, Paul Riesman (1992) describes two African societies where this notion is not present; there the child's personality is God-given, and as they grow up, their identity is shaped through their membership of and participation in the community and its culture.

6 This mother talked with us in the Risk Study. These comments have not been published elsewhere.

7 This father also talked with us in the Risk Study. His account has not been published elsewhere.

8 This excerpt has not been published elsewhere.

9 It should be acknowledged here that the siting and personnel participating in interviews make a difference to how people talk. Parents and children interviewed together at home in the Risk Study often put on a 'family front'; they protected the home and its social order from the interviewer. Conversations with children at school, especially with more than one child, tended to elicit more critical accounts of home life, some of this developed through participants confirming each others' comments (Kelley *et al.* 1997).

10 These comments by a mother in the Risk Study have not been published elsewhere.

11 Re Jane's mother's unaccompanied journeys to school at age 5, Newson and Newson, writing about 4-year-olds, indicate much more freedom to Nottingham young children in 1970 than is common in London now. For instance, they explain: 'At four he [*sic*] will rarely be allowed to wander unaccompanied more than a hundred yards or so from his own door, for fear of accident' (1970: 51). The Newsons refer to both traffic and stranger danger as self-evidently parents' two big fears (1978: 73, 95–7); but notably mothers of both 4- and 7-year-olds emphasize traffic rather than strangers as their reason for restricting children's explorations locally (Newson and Newson 1970: Ch. 3; 1978: Ch. 3).

12 Gudrun Ekstrand (1990), in a study of Swedish and Indian (Orissa) parents' understandings of child–adult relations, found that Indian parents assumed that children up to 16 years should obey and respect parents. Her work and other studies on parents' understandings are discussed by Gisela Eckert (2001).

Chapter 5 Childhood work

1 Christine Delphy (1984: 62, 96) uses the example of French farming households where the male head of the household expects unpaid labour from his younger sibs, his wife and his children, to make the more general point that patriarchy is alive and well. She refers to the *familia* – the Latin word for family – meaning all the land, slaves, women and children who are under the control of the father (1984: 62).

2 Miri Song (1997) describes children's work in Chinese takeaways as essential for family economic survival and as expected on the basis of family obligation.

3 Merryn Hutchings (1999) argues that children do regard some of their activities, including those at school, as work. It may be that the focus of her study – work (as contrasted with the focus of mine – daily life) somewhat accounts for differing findings. However, in common in the two studies is the point that the process of discussion with children tended to lead towards their recognition of school activity as work.

4 This section is not presented as a history of education (see, for example, Finch 1984; Gordon *et al.* 1991; Alexander 2000: Ch. 6).

5 Especially influential was the series of studies by Douglas, culminating in *The Home and the School* (1967), which gave new impetus to the parental involvement movement and to the identification of lower-class mothers as problems.

6 A *Guardian* article (18 April 2001) describes an organization which aims to improve children's school experience by modifying the buildings to make it more child-friendly.

7 See CHIPS Study (Mayall *et al.* 1996: 195–200). In children's accounts of the most recent illness episodes at school, two-fifths reported that their mother was summoned and came.

8 Case-study data from six schools in the CHIPS Study indicate that asthma, diabetes and epilepsy were among the commonest physical conditions facing teachers; in addition they described children with designated special needs (physical or behavioural). They also referred to other cases about which they were more sceptical. At a minimum estimate, based on teachers' reports, in 10 classes teachers had 34 children out of 264 (13 per cent; 3.4 per class on average) who had special needs for care (Mayall *et al.* 1996: 222).

9 A more recent empirical study (1996–8) provides similar data: variable SHS support and poor liaison between health and school staff; the authors stress the continuing need for clearer guidance and more systematic and effective school-based support (Lightfoot *et al.* 2001).

10 The accounts given by the class teacher and nurse at Town School have not previously been published. Hence no reference here to a publication and date.

11 Under Local Management of Schools initiatives, some of the financial resources for schools have been redistributed away from local authorities and directly to schools. Some have responded by appointing staff to manage the money.

12 The two classes concerned are Year 5 classes (children aged 9/10) in the Greenstreet Study (fieldwork 1990–1) and in the Childhood Study (1997–8).

13 In 1991, the first cohort of children aged 7, nationally, took the Key Stage 1 tests (Pollard *et al.* 1994). Tests at age 10/11 were established later in the 1990s (personal communication with Qualifications and Curriculum Authority).

14 Some figures: of the 28 9-year-olds at East Primary, 17 attended mosque each day after school, or a teacher came to their home. All the children had routine household duties. Twenty-six of the 28 attended some regular out-of-school activity once or more each week: sports, language classes, dance, music.

15 In the CHIPS Study case studies, children and teachers in two of the six schools told us of children's engagement with working up charters on school ethos, for children, staff and parents.

16 Homework assignments at this school are specifically addressed to child and parent/carer. The rationale is that this will educate the parent as well as involve them in their children's work. Some assignments can only be done if the parent participates. For instance, my 7-year-old granddaughter was asked to identify types of stone around the house and neighbourhood, to name them and say what they were used for. My 9-year-old grandson was asked to make a working robot.

When the homework policy was first implemented in the children's school, the children sometimes did not show assignments to their mother; mutual fury and recriminations – some directed at the school – ensued. Over time, both children and mother have accepted the unavoidable, and have modified home life accordingly.

17 Yet as I write, interactive processes have moved the agreement on. Resistance from the children, maternal exhaustion and joint irritation have served to postpone homework (again) to Sunday nights, at the last minute.

18 For discussion of Muslim girls' education in private and state secondary schools, see Haw 1998, especially Chapters 3 and 8, and Rassool 1999.

19 Stuart was in Year 8 at North Secondary School (Childhood Study). I arranged to talk with the young people in pairs, but he was busy with extra lessons, and then the class teacher suggested I talk with him on his own. I think she thought he might talk better so. In fact he simply told me his story (with little reference to my topic list).

20 For a recent analysis of children's schoolwork as work, see Qvortrup 2001.

21 There is some evidence that both poverty and minority ethnic status are implicated in how children and mothers deal with the attempts by education policies to engage the home in school activities. Ros Edwards (2000) reported more resistance to these policies among young people from 'working class circumstances' and from some minority ethnic groups to 'parental involvement', than among young people 'in middle class circumstances'. But we await detailed accounts of these intersections.

Chapter 6   The moral status of childhood

1 In this discussion, I am relying mainly on US scholars, who assume that the main site of early childhood is the nuclear family. This is a fair assumption for most UK childhoods too, but for other societies, the argument might range across wider kinship groups and the community (e.g. Riesman 1992; Woodhead *et al.* 1998).

2 It seems other societies and cultures recognize children's understanding of moral issues in early childhood. See von Hirsch 1998, for discussion of Jewish parents in Gateshead, England, and Eckert 2001: 18 for discussion of Arab Muslim and Christian parents in Sweden.

3 For discussion of mothers' appreciation of their children's moral engagement with family relations, in terms of both feelings and actions, see Brannen *et al.* 2000: Ch. 8. See also Mayall and Foster 1989: Ch. 2.

4 For discussion of how people shape events in their narratives, see Ribbens McCarthy *et al.* 2000.

5 For discussions, see Cullingford 1991: Ch. 7; Richards and Taylor 1998.

6 UK examples include: Chamberlin 1989; Meighan 1995; Meighan and Siraj-Blatchford 1997: Chapters 29–31; Osler 2000.

7 See Appendix (p. 192) for a note on the term 'Asian'.

8 Curfews for under-10s were introduced in 1998; and for under-16s in August 2001. However, the idea meets opposition on grounds of children's rights, community relations and practicality. It is thought no local authority has implemented these curfews (*Guardian*, 2 August 2001).

9 As suggested in Chapter 4 (p. 62) more recent studies are challenging the earlier assumption that teenagers wish to break away from their families. The issue of independence is intertwined with young people's sense of continuing responsibility towards their parents, and of interdependence. In a study of young people (aged 16–18) and their parents, mutual obligation and commitment shaped both groups' understandings of independence (Ribbens McCarthy 2001). For discussion of caring, with implications for children as carers, see also Mason 1996.

10 For discussion of arguments against the ascribed incompetence of children, see Verhellen 1993.

Chapter 7 Towards a child standpoint

1 Standpoint is a contentious topic within feminism, where people pointed out early on that to propose one standpoint was to prioritize white middle-class women; an uneasy consensus suggests the value of accepting varying standpoints, taking account of ethnicity and social class (see Ramazanoglu 1989; Alcoff and Potter 1993; Maynard 1994, 1998).

2 As Mead puts it: 'The social process, as involving communication, is in a sense responsible for the appearance of new objects in the field of experience of the individual organisms implicated in that process' (1967: 77).

3 For instance the sibling solidarity in E. Nesbit's books.

4 Recent studies on relations between sibs have indicated wide variation in their character (Dunn and McGuire 1992). Brannen et al. (2000: 116–18) also found variation, from antagonism to affection; but they also found evidence of 'support': learning from each other, caring about each other, friendship and confiding. Burke and Montgomery (2001) found that sibs of disabled children provided practical help, but also held a range of feelings about them.

5 In the CHIPS Study, the case-study schools with fewest complaints from children about bullying were County, which had large and varied playspaces, and Infant, where teachers organized and led games at play-time (Mayall et al. 1996: 184).

6 Play emerged spontaneously and so frequently in the Childhood Study, that later I (and friendly colleagues) explored it more formally with 20 children known to us (aged 6–12).

7 In parenthesis: young people also demonstrate (though do not refer to) another kind of play, as exemplified in 'the play of light'. Their conversations indicate how they play with ideas, skim across topics, delight in making jokes (see also Thorne 1993: 406).

8 Though there is a feminist literature, mainly from psychoanalytical points of view, which considers mothers' relations with their boy and girl children (for discussion, see Lawler 2000).

Chapter 8 Comparing childhoods

1 I gratefully acknowledge discussions with Leena Alanen during our work on these studies and her valuable contributions throughout this chapter. See also her paper on her study (Alanen 2001).

2 In Finland, those registered as unemployed, on parental leave (after the birth of a child) or on childcare leave (caring for an under-3 at home) are counted as employed.

3 Day nurseries are provided for children whose parents cannot or will not care for them. Some local authorities provide them free; others operate means-testing, but eligible parents mostly earn too little to be charged.

4 The childcare allowance allows parents to care for the child themselves or to organize childcare privately. It was introduced in part to encourage some parents to delay use of the expensive municipal daycare services.

5 Parents pay (on a means-tested basis) for daycare for pre-schoolers in Finland. Though compulsory – free – schooling starts at 7, 6-year-olds have been entitled to free pre-school education from August 2001.

6 Pringle (1998: 147) argues that the absence of solidaristic principles in the UK and USA allows for recognition of child abuse (and racism), in contrast to the Nordic countries. But it is difficult to substantiate a cause link.

7 Figures for 1991–5 show that, per 1000 children, traffic 'accidents' killed children: 2.9 (UK), 4.2 (Finland), 2.9 (Norway). Other injuries killed children: 3.2 (UK), 4.0 (Finland), 4.7 (Norway). All deaths from injury were 6.1 (UK), 8.2 (Finland) and 7.6 (Norway) (UNICEF 2001).

8 In order to ensure that lone parents – and their children – do not fall into poverty, they get financial support (reductions in daycare costs, tax reductions), with the effect that lone parent families are not much more likely than two-parent families to be in poverty. (In the 1990s recession, however, some of these supports were cut back.)

9 The UK fails on the percentage of women in parliament: 18 per cent, compared to Finland's 37 per cent (United Nations Development Fund for Women 2000: Table 3.3).

Chapter 9 Generation and gender

1 However, since detailed data on children's views of their moral status are not available from the past, we cannot say whether the current problems are new – probably not.

2 Among the many recent UK publications on children's rights are: Lansdown and Newell 1994; Save the Children 1995; Hodgkin and Newell 1996; Freeman 2000; Alderson 2000a; Lansdown 2001.

3 It is notable that while those who most need flexible working hours – women in the present inequitable division of labour – they are in practice less likely to have them than men (*Guardian*, 23 April 2001) – 52 per cent of all, 80 per cent of men, 52 per cent of women. Their interests are less well met than men's.

4 Recent reports discussing flexible work for parents in *The Guardian* include articles on 30 January 2001, 31 May 2001, 2 June 2001.

5 *The Guardian* newspaper asked schoolchildren to submit entries to a competition: The School We'd Like. 15,000 children in primary and secondary schools responded, some as individuals and some as classes (*Guardian*, 5 May 2001).

6 For a more recent analysis of the socioeconomic position of children worldwide and in the UK, together with wide-ranging suggestions for action, including revision of the CRC itself, see Freeman 2000.

7 Firestone (1971) and notably Christine Delphy (1984) took up Kate Millett's (1969) analysis of patriarchy and considered patriarchy in rural French families as it subjugates the male head of the household's dependants: both women and children. See Vinod Chandra's (2001) study of corner shop households (Ch. 5: 65).

8 I have trawled through recent publications, including Bradley (1996) and Ann Oakley's review of the literature (in preparation: Ch. 6); but cannot lay claim to have read everything in the vast outpouring of feminist work.

9 See Appendix (p. 191) for notes on usage of 'childcare' and 'daycare'.

10 A UNICEF paper (1998) arising from a 1998 conference with a worldwide focus on women's and children's rights, argues that perceived conflicts between them can be overcome by careful consideration of the issues affecting each group, and emphasizes that women and children have joint interests in 'shedding the burden of history' 'through creative strategies to overcome conservative appeals to culture, tradition, religion and customs' (1998: 12).

11 But, as I write, relationships between mothers' working and children's academic success have again been problematized in a research study which claims to have found poorer A-level results achieved by children whose mothers worked full-time in their pre-school years (*Guardian*, 14 March 2001; Ermisch and Francesconi 2001).

12 Daycare centres in Reggio Emilia have been one inspiration (Malaguzzi 1998). Here the underlying principle is that the daycare centre is a 'public forum situated in civil society, in which children and adults participate together in projects of social, cultural, political and economic significance' (Dahlberg *et al.* 1999: 73). More recently, Peter Moss (2001) and Helen Penn (2001) have reaffirmed their belief that what we need is neighbourhood centres for children of all ages, run democratically, with flexible hours to meet parental demand.

13 Feminist sociology of the family has also been slow to broaden its focus from preoccupation with adult relationships and divisions of labour, and from children as socialization projects, and towards analysis of child–adult relations where children are understood as agents (e.g. Silva and Smart 1999).

14 As noted in Chapter 6: 99, during the years of mainstream neglect of democratic working in schools, there has nevertheless been a steady stream of publications which keep the flag flying.

15 Priscilla Alderson examined this issue in her study of *Children's Consent to Surgery* (1993).

16 The UK government's second report to the United Nations on its progress towards implementing the CRC shows no sign of recognizing children's participation rights (United Kingdom 1999).

17 Dorothy Smith (quoted in Jaggar 1983: 386) notes: 'To begin from women's standpoint does not imply a common viewpoint among women. What we have in common is that organization of social relations which has accomplished our exclusion.'

Appendix

Four studies

I give here some details – in note form – about the four studies carried out in the 1990s, and which I use during this book. A brief description of the studies, including major findings, is given in Chapter 2.

The Greenstreet Study (1990–2)

Funded by the Nuffield Foundation and the Institute of Education, London University.
Researcher: Berry Mayall.
A small-scale study of children's ability to care for their own health at home and at school.
Samples: A reception class and a Year 5 class (4–6-year-olds and 9–10-year-olds) in one primary school in inner North London, with a mixed intake – by sex, social class and ethnicity. Numbers in the reception class rose during the fieldwork period from 22 to 25; there were 30 children in Class 5.

All the children wished to take part.

All parents of children in the two classes were asked if they were willing to be interviewed. Those who responded were listed randomly and approached in order of the list, keeping numbers of parents of boys and girls even. In the event, 12 parents of reception class and 10 of Year 5 were interviewed, with even number of parents of boys and girls. All the parents who made themselves available except two were mothers. These interviews took place at home, with the child present if s/he wished.

A class teacher of each year group (reception through to Class 6), the headteacher, school secretary and dinner ladies were also interviewed.

Fieldwork with the children included informal observation and conversations with children and teachers over two terms; more formal data collection was with pairs of children, whole class brainstorming, written work and drawings.

The principal themes discussed with all informants through conversations about children's daily lives at home and school were:

- the division of labour between mothers and school staff for children's health;
- the status of children's health at home and school;
- power relations between children, parents and teachers.

Main relevant publications: Mayall 1994, 1996.

The CHIPS Study (1993–5)

Applicants: Berry Mayall and Ann Oakley; 30 month study, funded by the Economic and Social Research Council; project reference number: ROOO 23 4476.
Researchers: Sandy Barker, Gill Bendelow, Berry Mayall, Pamela Storey and Marijke Veltman.
A study of the status of children's health in primary school.
Samples: A 1-in–20 random sample of schools in England and Wales were asked to complete an eight-sided postal questionnaire. The response rate was 60 per cent, number of completed questionnaires: 620.

After initial analysis of the questionnaire, case studies were carried out in six schools. These were chosen to include a range of types (infant, junior, all age); location: village, town, inner city, outer city; and area (London, midlands and the north of England).

The questionnaire, addressed to the headteacher, asked about:

- staff-child ratios;
- physical characteristics of the school;
- arrangements for maintaining and restoring children's health (meals, physical activity, sick rooms and trained staff);
- health education policy;
- the input of other agencies including the school health service.

The case studies addressed the same topics through interviews with headteachers, class teachers of Years 1 and 6, other staff (secretaries, PSE and PE coordinators, playground supervisors), the school nurse, parents of children in Years 1 and 6, and children in Years 1 and 6. In all there were 44 staff interviews, 112 responses from parents (including interviews and questionnaires), and data collected with 264 children (132 in each age-group). Data collection with the children focused also on their evaluation of the school, and their recent experiences of illness and accident at school.

Main relevant publications: Mayall *et al.* 1996; Mayall and Storey 1998.

The Risk Study (1995–6)

Applicants: Berry Mayall and Ann Oakley; 15-month study funded by the Economic and Social Research Council; project reference number: L211 25 2022, as one of 14 projects on the Risk and Human Behaviour Programme.

Researchers: Suzanne Hood, Peter Kelley and Berry Mayall.

This exploratory study considered children's and parents' views of the home as a place of risk or safety for children.

Samples: The study took place in a socially and ethnically mixed area of inner London. Samples were drawn from a general practitioner's list and from local schools. The sample included parents and children in 45 households and interviews were carried out with 59 parents at home, and with 27 9-year-olds (14 at home and 13 at school) and 21 12-year-olds (12 at home and 9 at a youth club). 20 3-year-olds were present at a parent interview and some contributed to the discussions.

The study explored with children and their parents their understandings of the home – as a place of risk or safety for children, in the context of other social settings – the neighbourhood and school. An open-ended topic list was used to encourage description and discussion of children's daily life at home. Themes in the research were:

- intergenerational identifications of risk;
- understandings of children and childhood;
- power relations between children and parents;
- how differing access to resources shapes children's and parents' understanding and management of risk.

Main relevant publications: Kelley *et al.* 1997, 1998.

The Childhood Study (1997–9)

Applicant: Berry Mayall, 24 month study, funded by the Economic and Social Research Council; project reference number L129 25 1032, as one of 22 projects on the Children 5–16 Programme.

Researchers: Berry Mayall and Helen Turner.

A study of children's agency in negotiating the character of their childhoods with parents and other important people in their lives.

Samples: The sample included 57 9-year-olds who comprised one Year 5 class at each of two primary schools in London: called East and North Primaries (Berry Mayall fieldwork). In addition, Helen Turner carried out paired discussions and individual interviews in a third primary school (called South Primary) with 15 9-year-olds; however these data are not referred to in this book, since I am much less familiar with them.

Secondary schools were then chosen on the basis that many of the children from the East and North Primary Schools go to them; data were collected with young people in Year 8 (aged 12–13): 37 at an East girls secondary and a mixed secondary, and 30 at a North mixed secondary.

At North schools, the children were socially and ethnically mixed. At East schools, most of the children were from ethnic minorities, including substantial proportions whose family's origins were in the Indian subcontinent.

Access to the primary school children was unproblematic; the class teachers were cooperative, parental consent not a problem and all the children agreed. Fieldwork took place in each class over the course of one term, one or two days a week.

Access to the East Secondary School students was more problematic; not all parents returned consent forms; staff allowed only one session with each student. Helen Turner and I, separately, held paired single-sex discussions with girls and boys, and also two group discussions with girls.

Access in North Secondary was as in the primary schools: parents agreed and staff were happy for extended contact over one term, all but one of the students wished to take part; fieldwork included paired interviews, individual interviews, group discussions and informal participant observation (Berry Mayall fieldwork).

The principal topics explored with all the young people were:

- their understandings of the social status of childhood and parenthood;
- processes in child–adult relations;
- their experiences of and reflections on their daily lives – with emphasis on their lives out of school.

Main relevant publications: Mayall 2000, 2001.

Notes on research with children

Research with children has come a long way since the early 90s. People are finding that it can be done, and with younger and younger children, and they have devised a range of methods to do this work (e.g. Waksler 1991; Sinclair 1996; Hart 1997; Johnson *et al.* 1998; Christensen and James 2000; Clark and Moss 2001; and papers in many issues of the journals *Childhood* and *Children and Society*). In this book I have not spent a great deal of space discussing methods, relations between the researcher and the researched, the status of children's accounts or issues of interpretation. How to represent voices is an important area for study (Alldred 1998), but to do it well demands all the space there is. In this book, instead, I have given space to extended extracts from children's accounts so that they speak for themselves. My main aim has been to develop an argument towards a sociology of childhood and to use empirical data as a means to that end. I think I use data in the following somewhat distinct ways:

- to *illustrate, exemplify* points previously discovered in analysis. Thus I quote in order to illustrate how children's accounts reflect macro points, for instance on traffic policy, in talking about constraints on their own lives (Chapter 4: 58). I give examples of the ways children talk about rights (Chapter 6: 98). In Chapter 4, I give summary case studies to exemplify differences between childhoods;
- to *demonstrate*. Here the aim is to give a sound basis for making a point. Sometimes I use long passages so that readers can see for themselves how children construct arguments, refine points, show conflicting ideas. An example here is the long excerpt from Sandra's account of an episode in her life, which demonstrates the complexity of her moral engagement with the issues it raised for her (Chapter 6: 90). Another example of demonstration is excerpts from group discussions, which show how a group constitutes childhood through refining points with each other (Chapter 7: 123). And a third example is where quotations show how

children, asked about the importance of play in their lives, link their answers to the notion of 'free time' and its definition as time out of adult control (Chapter 7: 134);

- to *discuss issues* through detailed consideration of the data. Here I mean that accounts can be scanned across one child's or several children's accounts in order to discuss what they seem to reveal (to me in my ivory tower). For instance, in Chapter 5 (83) I discuss the extent to which a child's account points to his participation in intermediate domain work; this concept is not part of the child's understanding of his agency, but for the onlooker it is useful for analysing the account. Another example is the use of several differing accounts of the nature of 'work', which are used to discuss work as a constituent part of childhood activity (Chapter 5: 66).

In part, I use quotations from children as one means of presenting their views. A common concern among researchers has been that adults cannot adequately represent children's views; and quotation does at least bring into the equation the actual words they use and the ways their discussions with each other proceed. But the analysis, conceptualizing and writing up do take place at a distance from those words and do give a shape to them that they might not agree with. The adult researcher's work with young people is, I think, comparable to her work with women, since analysis, categorizing and writing up at a distance from actual people and in an ivory tower, is common to both enterprises. These enterprises are undertaken by people whose relation to the social order commonly differs from that of the people researched.

Please note that all names assigned to schools and to children are pseudonyms.

Terms

'Child'

In dealing with the term 'child', I have tried to distinguish between usages according to context. 'Child' is both social status in relation and contradistinction to adulthood and it is a kinship term (I am still my mother's child). I use the term 'child' when the context is its relational or kinship meaning. Many discussions in this book are about accounts of childhood given by people who adult onlookers may assume belong to the same category; that is we are dealing with 'children's' accounts of childhood. So it was important to distinguish between my informants and their topic. Young people offered many definitions of 'child'. These included legal understandings; for instance the UN Convention on the Rights of the Child defines under-18s as children. They often distinguished between social stages – baby, toddler, child, teenager – or between social statuses: children at primary school and students at secondary school. They also defined 'child' in contradistinction to 'adult'. So where I am discussing with young people their definitions or characteristics of childhood, I describe my informants as 'young people' in order to indicate that they may or may not site themselves within the category 'child', and that 'child' is a problematic category.

'Childcare' and 'daycare'

When discussing adults' care of children, I use 'childcare' for care by any adult, including parents, and 'daycare' to mean services provided by non-parents.

'Asian'

Common UK usage, currently, is to refer to people whose family origins are in India, Pakistan and Bangladesh as 'Asian'. The 2001 National Census did so (National Statistics 2001). Young people in the Childhood Study commonly referred to themselves and friends as Asian. Issues around this designation are discussed by Alibhai-Brown (2000: ix–xiii). Wherever possible I avoid this designation, but do occasionally use it, for shorthand.

References

Abrams, P. (1982) *Historical Sociology*. Shepton Mallet: Open Books.

Adonis, A. and Pollard, S. (1997) *The Myth of Britain's Classless Society*. Harmondsworth: Penguin.

Alanen, L. (1988) Rethinking childhood, *Acta Sociologica*, 31: 53–67.

Alanen, L. (1992) *Modern Childhood? Exploring the 'Child Question' in Sociology*. Research Report 50. Finland: University of Jyväskylä.

Alanen, L. (1996) Social policy and generational relations: child policy in a Nordic landscape. Paper presented at colloquium: Politics for Children, with Children or against Children, Munich: Deutsches Jugendinstitut, May.

Alanen, L. (1998) Children and the family order, in I. Hutchby and J. Moran-Ellis (eds) *Children and Social Competence*. London: Falmer.

Alanen, L. (2000) From sociologies of childhood to generational analysis. Paper presented at seminar Childhood and Social Theory, University of Keele, 13–14 April.

Alanen, L. (2001) Explorations in generational analysis, in L. Alanen and B. Mayall (eds) *Conceptualizing Child-Adult Relations*. London: RoutledgeFalmer.

Alanen, L. and Bardy, M. (1990) *Childhood as a Social Phenomenon: National Report Finland*. Eurosocial Report 36/7. Vienna: European Centre.

Alcoff, L. and Potter, E. (1993) *Feminist Epistemologies*. London: Routledge.

Alderson, P. (1993) *Children's Consent to Surgery*. Buckingham: Open University Press.

Alderson, P. (1999a) Human rights and democracy in schools – do they mean more than 'picking up litter and not killing whales'? *International Journal of Children's Rights*, 7: 185–205.

Alderson, P. (1999b) *Civil Rights in Schools*. Children 5–16 Research Briefing No. 1. Swindon: Economic and Social Research Council.

Alderson, P. (2000a) *Young Children's Rights: Exploring Beliefs, Principles and Practice*. London: Jessica Kingsley.

Alderson, P. (2000b) Children as researchers: The effects of participation rights on research methodology, in P. Christensen and A. James (eds) *Research with Children: Perspectives and Practices*. London: RoutledgeFalmer.

Alderson, P. (2000c) Citizenship in theory and practice: Being or becoming citizens with rights, in D. Lawton, J. Cairns and R. Gardner (eds) *Education for Citizenship*. London: Continuum.

Alderson, P. and Goodey, C. (1998) *Enabling Education: Experiences in Special and Ordinary Schools*. London: Tufnell Press.

Aldridge, J. and Becker, S. (1995) The rights and wrongs of children who care, in B. Franklin (ed.) *The Handbook of Children's Rights: Comparative Policy and Practice*. London: Routledge.

Alexander, R. (2000) *Culture and Pedagogy: International Comparisons in Primary Education*. Oxford: Blackwell.

Alibhai-Brown, Y. (2000) *Who Do We Think We Are?* Harmondsworth: The Penguin Press.

Allatt, P. (1996) Conceptualizing parenting from the standpoint of children: Relationship and transition in the life course, in J. Brannen and M. O'Brien (eds) *Children in Families: Research and Policy*. London: Falmer.

Alldred, P. (1998) Ethnography and discourse analysis: dilemmas in representing the voice of children, in J. Ribbens and R. Edwards (eds) *Feminist Dilemmas in Qualitative Research: Public Knowledge and Private Lives*. London: Sage.

Alldred, P., David, M. and Edwards, R. (2002) Minding the gap: Children and young people negotiating relations between home and school, in R. Edwards (ed.) *Children, Home and School: Autonomy, Connection or Regulation*. London: RoutledgeFalmer.

Apple, M. and Beane, J. (1999) *Democratic Schools: Lessons from the Chalk Face*. Buckingham: Open University Press.

Appleton, P. (1995) Young people with disability: aspects of social empowerment, in C. Cloke and M. Davies (eds) *Participation and Empowerment in Child Protection*. Chichester: John Wiley.

Archer, M. (1982) Morphogenesis versus structuration. *British Journal of Sociology*, 33: 455–83.

Archer, M. (1998) Social theory and the analysis of society, in T. May and M. Williams (eds) *Knowing the Social World*. Buckingham: Open University Press.

Bacchi, C.L. (1999) *Women, Policy and Politics: The Construction of Policy Problems*. London: Sage.

Barrett, M. and McIntosh, M. (1982) *The Anti-social Family*. London: Verso.

Barry, M. (2001) *Young People's Views and Experiences of Growing Up*. JRF Findings. York: Joseph Rowntree Foundation.

Beck, U. (1992) *Risk Society*. London: Sage.

Bendelow, G. and Mayall, B. (2000) How children manage emotions in schools, in S. Fineman (ed.) *Emotions in Organizations*. London: Sage.

Bentley, T. (1998) *Learning Beyond the Classroom: Education for a Changing World*. London: Routledge.

Bhachu, P. (1993) Identities constructed and reconstructed: Representations of Asian women in Britain, in G. Buijs (ed.) *Migrant Women: Crossing Ethnic Boundaries and Changing Identities*. Oxford: Berg.

Bhaskar, R. (1979) *The Possibility of Naturalism*. Brighton: Harvester Press.

du Bois-Reymond, M., Büchner, P. and Krüger, H.H. (1993) Modern family as everyday negotiation: Continuities and discontinuities in parent–child relationships, *Childhood*, 1(2): 87–99.

Bottomore, T.B. and Rubel, M. (eds) (1963) *Karl Marx: Selected Writings in Sociology and Social Philosophy*. Harmondsworth: Penguin.

Bourdieu, P. (1986) The forms of capital, in J. Richardson (ed.) *Handbook of Theory and Research for the Sociology of Education*. New York: Greenwood.

Bourdieu, P. (1988) *Homo Academicus*. Cambridge: Polity Press.

Bourdieu, P. (1993) A science that makes trouble, in P. Bourdieu, *Sociology in Question*. London: Sage.

Bowlby, J. (1953) *Child Care and the Growth of Love*. Harmondsworth: Penguin.

Boyden, J. (1997) Childhood and the policy-makers: a comparative perspective on the globalization of childhood, in A. James and A. Prout (eds) *Constructing and Reconstructing Childhood: Contemporary Issues in the Sociological Study of Childhood*. London: Falmer.

Bradley, H. (1996) *Fractured Identities: Changing Patterns of Inequality*. Cambridge: Polity Press.

Brannen, J. (1996) Discourses of adolescence: Young people's independence and autonomy within families, in J. Brannen and M. O'Brien (eds) *Children in Families: Research and Policy*. London: Falmer Press.

Brannen, J., Heptinall, E. and Bhopal, K. (2000) *Connecting Children: Care and Family Life in Later Childhood*. London: RoutledgeFalmer.

Bruner, J. (1990) *Acts of Meaning*. Cambridge, MA: Harvard University Press.

Bruner, J., Jolly, H. and Sylva, K. (eds) (1976) *Play: Its Role in Development and Evolution*. Harmondsworth: Penguin.

Bryson, L., Bittman, M. and Donath, S. (1994) Men's welfare state, women's welfare state: Tendencies to convergence in practice and theory? in D. Sainsbury (ed.) *Gendering Welfare States*. London: Sage.

Bryson, V. (1999) *Feminist Debates: Issues of Theory and Political Practice*. London: Macmillan.

Buckingham, D. (2000) *After the Death of Childhood: Growing Up in the Age of Electronic Media*. Cambridge: Polity.

Burke, P. and Montgomery, S. (2001) *Finding a Voice: Supporting the Brothers and Sisters of Children with Disabilities*. Hull: Department of Social Work, University of Hull.

Burman, E. (1994) *Deconstructing Developmental Psychology*. London: Routledge.

Burns, A. (1995) Mother-headed families: Here to stay? in J. Brannen and M. O'Brien (eds) *Childhood and Parenthood*. Proceedings of a conference, Childhood and Parenthood, April. London: Institute of Education.

Cahill, S. (1990) Childhood and public life: reaffirming biographical divisions, *Social Problems*, 37(3): 390–401.

Campbell, J. (1998) Primary teaching: Roles and relationships, in C. Richards and P.H. Taylor (eds) *How Shall We School Our Children? Primary Education and its Future*. London: Falmer.

Candappa, M. (2000a) *Extraordinary Childhoods: The Social Lives of Refugee*

Children. Research Briefing No. 5. Swindon: Economic and Social Research Council.

Candappa, M. (2000b) Building a new life: The role of the school in supporting refugee children, *Multi-cultural Teaching*, 19(1): 28–32.

Carter, C. (2000) Meeting the challenge of inclusion: Human rights education to improve relationships in a boys' school, in A. Osler (ed.) *Citizenship and Democracy in Schools: Diversity, Identity, Equality*. Stoke on Trent: Trentham Books.

Central Advisory Council for Education (England) (1967) *Children and Their Primary Schools* (Plowden Report) vol. 1. London: HMSO.

Chamberlin, R. (1989) *Free Children and Democratic Schools: A Philosophical Study of Liberty and Education*. London: Falmer Press.

Chandra, V. (2001) Children's work in the family: a sociological study of Indian children in Coventry (UK) and Lucknow (India). Unpublished PhD thesis, University of Warwick.

Children's Rights Development Unit (CRDU) (1994) *UK Agenda for Children*. London: CRDU.

Christensen, P. and James, A. (eds) (2000) *Research with Children: Perspectives and Practices*. London: RoutledgeFalmer.

Christensen, P. and James, A. (2001) What are schools for? The temporal experience of children's learning in northern England, in L. Alanen and B. Mayall (eds) *Conceptualising Child–Adult Relations*. London: Falmer.

Clark, A. and Moss, P. (2001) *Listening to Young Children: The Mosaic Approach*. London: National Children's Bureau.

Cockburn, T. (1998) Children and citizenship in Britain, *Childhood*, 5(1): 99–118.

Cole, M. (1996) *Cultural Psychology*. Cambridge, MA: Harvard University Press.

Connell, R. (1987) *Gender and Power*. Cambridge: Polity Press.

Corsaro, W. (1996) *The Sociology of Childhood*. Thousand Oaks, CA: Pine Forge Press.

Corsten, M. (1999) The time of generations, *Time and Society*, 8(2): 249–72.

Cowan, R., Traill, D. and McNaughton, S. (1998) Homework for primary school-children: Ideals and reality, *The Psychology of Education Review*, 22(2): 20–7.

Craib, I. (1992) *Modern Social Theory: From Parsons to Habermas*. Brighton: Harvester Wheatsheaf.

Cronin, N., McGlone, F. and Millar, J. (1996) United Kingdom, in J. Ditch, H. Barnes, H. and J. Bradshaw (eds) *Developments in National Family Policies in 1995*. York: Social Policy Research Unit.

Cullingford, C. (1991) *The Inner World of the School: Children's Ideas about Schools*. London: Cassell.

Cunningham, H. (1991) *The Children of the Poor: Representations of Childhood since the Seventeenth Century*. Oxford: Blackwells.

Cunningham, J. (2000) Democratic practice in a secondary school, in A. Osler (ed.) *Citizenship and Democracy in Schools: Diversity, Identity, Equality*. Stoke on Trent: Trentham Books.

Dahlberg, G., Moss, P. and Pence, A. (1999) *Beyond Quality in Early Childhood Education and Care: Post-Modern Perspectives*. London: Falmer Press.

Damon, W. (1990) *The Moral Child: Nurturing Children's Natural Moral Growth*. New York: The Free Press.

David, M., Edwards, R., Hughes, M. and Ribbens, J. (1993) *Mothers and Education: Inside Out?* London: Macmillan.

David, M., Weiner, G. and Arnot, M. (1997) Strategic feminist research on gender equality and schooling in Britain in the 1990s, in C. Marshall (ed.) *Feminist Critical Policy Analysis I: A Perspective from Primary and Secondary Schooling.* London: Falmer.

Davies, M. and Cloke, C. (1995) Introduction, in C. Cloke and M. Davies (eds) *Participation and Empowerment in Child Protection.* Chichester: John Wiley.

Davin, A. (1990) When is a child not a child? in H. Corr and L. Jamieson (eds) *Politics of Everyday Life.* London: Macmillan.

Dearden, C., Becker, S. and Aldridge, J. (1994) *Partners in Caring: A Briefing for Professionals about Young Carers.* Loughborough: Loughborough University Young Carers Research Group.

Delanty, G. (1997) *Social Science: Beyond Constructivism and Realism.* Buckingham: Open University Press.

Delphy, C. (1984) *Close to Home: A Materialist Analysis of Women's Oppression.* London: Hutchinson.

Department for Education and Employment (1998) *Home–School Agreements: Guidance for Schools.* London: DfEE.

Douglas, J.W.B. (1967) *The Home and the School.* London: Panther Books.

Dunn, J. (1984) *Sisters and Brothers.* London: Fontana Books.

Dunn, J. (1988) *The Beginnings of Social Understanding.* Oxford: Blackwells.

Dunn, J. and McGuire, J. (1992) Sibling and peer relationships in childhood, *Journal of Child Psychology and Psychiatry*, 33(1): 67–105.

Durkheim, E. (1961) *Moral Education: A Study in the Theory and Application of the Sociology of Education.* New York: Free Press of Glencoe (first published 1912).

Eckert, G. (2001) *Wasting Time or Having Fun: Cultural Meanings of Children and Childhood.* Linköping, Sweden: Faculty of Arts and Sciences, Linköping University.

Edwards, C.P. (1986) Culture and the construction of moral values: A comparative ethnography of moral encounters in two cultural settings, in J. Kagan and S. Lamb (eds) *The Emergence of Morality in Young Children.* Chicago, IL: University of Chicago Press.

Edwards, R. (2000) *Children's Understandings of Parental Involvement in Education.* Children 5–16 Research Briefing No. 11. Swindon: Economic and Social Research Council.

Edwards, R. and Alldred, P. (2000) A typology of parental involvement in education centring on children and young people: negotiating familialisation, institutionalisation and individualisation, *British Journal of Sociology of Education*, 21(3): 435–55.

Ekstrand, G. (1990) *Culture's Children: Comparative Analyses of Cultural Patterns Regarding Conditions for Children and Youth in Sweden and Orissa.* Stockholm: Almqvist and Wiksell International.

Elshtain, J.B. (1981) *Public Man, Private Woman: Women in Social and Political Thought.* Princeton, NJ: Princeton University Press.

Engelbert, A. (1994) Worlds of childhood: Differentiated but different. Implications for social policy, in J. Qvortrup, M. Bardy, G. Sgritta and H. Wintersberger (eds) *Childhood Matters: Social Theory, Practice and Politics*. Aldershot: Avebury Press.

Ennew, J. (1986) *The Sexual Exploitation of Children*. Cambridge: Polity Press.

Ennew, J. (1994) *Childhood as a Social Phenomenon: National Report England and Wales*. Eurosocial Report 36/16. Vienna: European Centre.

Erikson, E. (1968) *Identity, Youth and Crisis*. London: Faber and Faber.

Ermisch, J. and Francesconi, M. (2001) *The Effect of Parents' Employment on Outcomes for Children*. JRF Findings. York: Joseph Rowntree Foundation.

Finch, J. (1984) *Education as Social Policy*. London: Longman.

Firestone, S. (1971) *The Dialectics of Sex*. London: Jonathan Cape.

Franklin, B. (1995) The case for children's rights: A progress report, in B. Franklin (ed.) *The Handbook of Children's Rights*. London: Routledge.

Freeman, M. (2000) The future of children's rights, *Children and Society*, 14(4): 277–93.

Freire, P. (1996) *Pedagogy of the Oppressed*. Harmondsworth: Penguin.

Frønes, I., Jensen, A.-M. and Solberg, A. (1990) *Childhood as a Social Phenomenon: National Report Norway*. Eurosocial Report 36/1. Vienna: European Centre.

Gavron, K. (1997) Migrants to citizens: Changing orientations among Bangladeshis of Tower Hamlets, London. Unpublished PhD thesis, London University.

Ghate, D. and Daniels, A. (1997) *Talking about my Generation*. London: NSPCC.

Giddens, A. (1979) *Central Problems in Social Theory*. London: Macmillan.

Giddens, A. (1984) *The Constitution of Society*. Cambridge: Polity Press.

Giddens, A. (1991) *Modernity and Self-Identity: Self and Society in the Late Modern Age*. Cambridge: Polity Press.

Gill, T. (2001) Editorial. *Play Today*, Issue 23, February, p. 2.

Goffman, I. (1968) *Asylums*. Harmondsworth: Penguin.

Gordon, P., Aldrich, R. and Dean, D. (1991) *Education and Policy in England in the Twentieth Century*. London: Woburn Press.

Gordon, T., Holland, J. and Lahelma, E. (2000) *Making Spaces: Citizenship and Difference in Schools*. London: Macmillan.

Graham, H. (1983) Caring: A labour of love, in J. Finch and D. Groves (eds) *A Labour of Love: Women, Work and Caring*. London: Routledge and Kegan Paul.

Green, A. (1990) *Education and State Formation: The Rise of Education Systems in England, France and the USA*. London: Macmillan.

Green, A. (1997) *Education, Globalization and the Nation State*. London: Macmillan.

Griffith, A. (1995) Mothering, schooling and children's devleopment, in M. Campbell and A. Manicom (eds) *Knowledge, Experience and Ruling Relations*. Toronto: University of Toronto Press.

Hammersley, M. and Atkinson, P. (1983) *Ethnography: Principles and Practice*. London: Tavistock.

Harding, S. (1991) *Whose Science? Whose Knowledge? Thinking from Women's Lives*. Buckingham: Open University Press.

Hardyment, C. (1983) *Dream Babies: Child Care from Locke to Spock*. Oxford: Oxford University Press.

Harré, R. (1986) The step to social constructionism, in M. Richards and P. Light (eds) *Children of Social Worlds*. Cambridge: Polity.

Harris, B. (1995) *The Health of the Schoolchild: A History of the School Medical Service in England and Wales*. Buckingham: Open University Press.

Hart, R. (1997) *Children's Participation: The Theory and Practice of Involving Young Citizens in Community Development and Environmental Care*. London: Earthscan Publications Ltd.

Hartsock, N. (1983) The feminist standpoint: Developing the ground for a specifically feminist historical materialism, in S. Harding and M. Hintikka (eds) *Discovering Reality: Feminist Perspectives on Epistemology, Metaphysics, Methodology, and Philosophy of Science*. Dordrecht: D. Reidel Publishing Company.

Haw, K. (1998) *Educating Muslim Girls*. Buckingham: Open University Press.

Hendrick, H. (1994) *Child Welfare, England 1872–1989*. London: Routledge.

Hendrick, H. (1997) Constructions and reconstructions of British childhood: An interpretative survey, 1800 to the present, in A. James and A. Prout (eds) *Constructing and Reconstructing Childhood: Contemporary Issues in the Sociological Study of Childhood*, 2nd edn. London: Falmer.

Highfield Junior School (1997) *Changing Our School: Promoting Positive Behaviour*. Highfield School and London: Institute of Education.

Hillman, M. (1993) One false move: A study of children's independent mobility, in M. Hillman (ed.) *Children, Transport and the Quality of Life*. London: Policy Studies Institute.

Hodgkin, R. and Newell, P. (1996) *Effective Government Structures for Children*. Report of a Gulbenkian Foundation Inquiry. London: Calouste Gulbenkian Foundation.

Holland, J. and Blair, M. with Sheldon, S. (eds) (1995) *Debates and Issues in Feminist Research and Pedagogy*. Buckingham: Open University Press.

Hood, S. (1999) Home–school agreements: a true partnership? *School Leadership and Management*, 19(4): 427–40.

Hood, S. (2001) *The State of London Children's Report*. London: Office of the Children's Rights Commissioner for London.

Hood-Williams, J. (1990) Patriarchy for children: On the stability of power relations in children's lives, in L. Chisholm, P. Büchner, H.-H. Krüger, and P. Brown (eds) *Childhood, Youth and Social Change: A Comparative Perspective*. London: Falmer Press.

House of Commons (1997) *Health Services for Children and Young People in the Community: Home and School*. Third report of the Health Committee. London: HMSO.

Hughes, M., Mayall, B., Moss, P. *et al.* (1980) *Nurseries Now: A Fair Deal for Parents and Children*. Harmondsworth: Penguin.

Huizinga, J. (1949) *Homo Ludens: A Study of the Play-Element in Culture*. London: Routledge and Kegan Paul.

Humphries, S. and Rowe, S. (1994) The biggest classroom, in P. Blatchford and S. Sharp (eds) *Breaktime and the School: Understanding and Changing Playground Behaviour*. London: Routledge.

Hurt, J.S. (1979) *Elementary Schooling and the Working Classes 1860–1918*. London: Routledge.

Husain, F. and O'Brien, M. (1998) *South Asian Muslims in Britain: Faith, Family and Community*. London: Department of Environmental and Social Studies, University of North London.

Hutchby, I. and Moran-Ellis, J. (1998) Siting children's social competence, in I. Hutchby and J. Moran-Ellis (eds) *Children and Social Competence: Arenas of Action*. London: Falmer.

Hutchby, I. and Moran-Ellis, J. (eds) (2001) *Children, Technology and Culture: The Impacts of Technologies in Children's Everyday Lives*. London: RoutledgeFalmer.

Hutchings, M. (1999) Children's constructions of work: Transfer of ideas between different work contexts. Paper presented to the Sites of Learning Conference, University of Hull, September.

Hutt, S.J., Tyler, S., Hutt, C. and Christopherson, D. (1989) *Play, Exploration and Learning*. London: Routledge.

Ingleby, D. (1986) Development in social context, in M. Richards and P. Light (eds) *Children of Social Worlds*. Cambridge: Polity.

Jaggar, A.M. (1983) *Feminist Politics and Human Nature*. Brighton, Sussex: Harvester Press.

James, A. (1998) Play in childhood: An anthropological perspective, *Child Psychology and Psychiatry Review*, 3(3): 104–12.

James, A., Jenks, C. and Prout, A. (1998) *Theorising Childhood*. London: Polity.

James, A. and James, A. (2001) Tightening the net: Children, community and control, *British Journal of Sociology*, 52(2): 211–28.

James, A. and Prout, A. (eds) (1997) *Constructing and Reconstructing Childhood: Contemporary Issues in the Sociological Study of Childhood*. London: Falmer.

Jenks, C. (ed.) (1982) *The Sociology of Childhood*. London: Batsford.

Jenks, C. (1996) *Childhood*. London: Routledge.

Jensen, A.-M. (1994) The feminisation of childhood, in J. Qvortrup, M. Bardy, G. Sgritta and H. Wintersberger (eds) *Childhood Matters: Social Theory, Practice and Politics*. Aldershot: Avebury Press.

Johnson, V., Ivan-Smith, E., Gordon, G., Pridmore, P. and Scott, P. (1998) *Stepping Forward: Children and Young People's Participation in the Development Process*. London: Intermediate Technology Publications.

Kagan, J. (1986) Introduction, in J. Kagan and S. Lamb (eds) *The Emergence of Morality in Young Children*. Chicago, IL: University of Chicago Press.

Kagitcibasi, C. (1996) *Family and Human Development: A View from the Other Side*. Hove: Lawrence Erlbaum.

Kartovaara, L. and Sauli, H. (2000) *The Finnish Child: Official Statistics of Finland, Population 2000: 7*. Helsinki: Statistics Finland.

Kelley, P., Hood, S. and Mayall, B. (1998) Children, parents and risk, *Health and Social Care in the Community*, 6(1): 16–24.

Kelley, P., Mayall, B. and Hood, S. (1997) Children's accounts of risk, *Childhood*, 4(3): 305–24.

Kiddle, C. (1998) *Traveller Children: A Voice for Themselves*. London: Jessica Kingsley Publishers.

Kline, S. (2001) Children and media – in the age of marketing. Papers from a conference: Children's Living Conditions and Welfare, Vedbaek, Denmark, 20–21 November 2000.

Knutsson, K.E. (1997) *Children: Noble Causes or Worthy Citizens*. Florence, Italy: United Nations Children's Fund.

Kvist, J. (1999) Welfare reform in the Nordic countries in the 1990s: Using fuzzy-set theory to assess conformity to ideal types, *Journal of European Social Policy*, 9(3): 231–52.

La Fontaine, J. (1999) Are children people? in J. La Fontaine and H. Rydström (eds) *The Invisibility of Children*. Working papers on childhood and the study of children. Department of Child Studies, University of Linköping, Sweden.

Langford, W., Lewis, C., Solomon, Y. and Warin, J. (2001) *Closeness, Authority and Independence in Families with Teenagers*. York: Joseph Rowntree Foundation.

Lansdown, G. (1995) The Children's Rights Development Unit, in B. Franklin (ed.) *The Handbook of Children's Rights*. London: Routledge.

Lansdown, G. (2001) *Promoting Children's Participation in Democratic Decision-making*. Florence, Italy: UNICEF.

Lansdown, G. and Newell, P. (1994) *UK Agenda for Children*. London: Children's Rights Development Unit.

Lawler, S. (2000) *Mothering the Self: Mothers, Daughters, Subjects*. London: Routledge.

Layder, D. (1994) *Understanding Social Theory*. London: Sage.

Layder, D. (1997) *Modern Social Theory: Key Debates and New Directions*. London: UCL Press.

Layder, D. (1998a) *Sociological Practice: Linking Theory and Social Research*. London: Sage.

Layder, D. (1998b) The reality of social domains: Implications for theory and method, in T. May and M. Williams (eds) *Knowing the Social World*. Buckingham: Open University Press.

Leach, P. (1979) *Who Cares: A New Deal for Mothers and Their Small Children*. Harmondsworth: Penguin.

Lee, N. (2001) *Childhood and Society*. Buckingham: Open University Press.

Leira, A. (1998) Caring as a social right: Cash for child care and daddy leave, *Social Politics*, 5(3): 362–78.

Leonard, D. (1990) Persons in their own right: Children and sociology in the UK, in L. Chisholm, P. Büchner, H.-H. Krüger and P. Brown (eds) *Childhood, Youth and Social Change: A Comparative Perspective*. London: Falmer Press.

Lightfoot, J., Mukherjee, S. and Sloper, P. (2001) Supporting pupils with special health needs in mainstream schools: Policy and practice, *Children and Society*, 15(2): 57–69.

Lindley, R. (1989) Teenagers and other children, in G. Scarre (ed.) *Children, Parents and Politics*. Cambridge: Cambridge University Press.

Little, J., Peake, L. and Richardson, P. (eds) (1988) *Women in Cities: Gender and the Urban Environment*. London: Macmillan Education.

Maclachlan, K. (1996) Good mothers are women too: The gender implications of parental involvement in education, in J. Bastiani and S. Wolfendale (eds) *Home–School Work in Britain*. London: David Fulton Publishers.

Malaguzzi, L. (1998) History, ideas and basic philosophy: An interview with Lella Gandini, in C. Edwards, L. Gandini and G. Forman (eds) *The Hundred Lan-*

guages of Children: The Reggio Emilia Approach – Advanced Reflections. 2nd edn. Greenwich, CT: Ablex Publishing Corporation.

Manicom, A. (1995) What's health got to do with it? Class, gender and teachers' work, in M. Campbell and A. Manicom (eds) *Knowledge, Experience and Ruling Relations: Studies in the Social Organisation of Knowledge.* Toronto: University of Toronto Press.

Mannheim, K. (1952) The problem of generations, in K. Mannheim, *Essays on the Sociology of Knowledge.* London: Routledge and Kegan Paul (first published in 1928).

Martin, E. (1989) *The Woman in the Body.* Buckingham: Open University Press.

Marx, K. and Engels, F. (1970) *The German Ideology.* London: Lawrence and Wishart.

Mason, J. (1996) Gender, care and sensibility in family and kin relationships, in J. Holland and L. Adkins (eds) *Sex, Sensibility and the Gendered Body.* Explorations in Sociology 46. London: Macmillan/British Sociological Association.

Matthews, G.B. (1980) *Philosophy and the Young Child.* Cambridge, MA: Harvard University Press.

Matthews, G.B. (1984) *Dialogues with Children.* Cambridge, MA: Harvard University Press.

Matthews, G.B. (1994) *The Philosophy of Childhood.* Cambridge, MA: Harvard University Press.

Matthews, H., Taylor, M., Percy-Smith, B. and Limb, M. (2000) The unacceptable *flaneur*: The shopping mall as a teenage hangout, *Childhood*, 7(3): 279–94.

Mayall, B. (1981) Childminding as a service for working mothers and their children aged under two years. Unpublished PhD thesis, University of London.

Mayall, B. (1986) *Keeping Children Healthy.* London: Allen & Unwin.

Mayall, B. (1993) Keeping children healthy – the intermediate domain, *Social Science and Medicine*, 36(1): 77–84.

Mayall, B. (1994) *Negotiating Health: Children at Home and Primary School.* London: Cassell.

Mayall, B. (1996) *Children, Health and the Social Order.* Buckingham: Open University Press.

Mayall, B. (2000) The sociology of childhood in relation to children's rights, *International Journal of Children's Rights*, 8: 243–59.

Mayall, B. (2001) Understanding childhoods: A London study, in L. Alanen and B. Mayall (eds) *Conceptualizing Child–Adult Relations.* London: Falmer Press.

Mayall, B., Bendelow, G., Barker, S., Storey, P. and Veltman, M. (1996) *Children's Health in Primary Schools.* London: Falmer.

Mayall, B. and Foster, M.-C. (1989) *Child Health Care: Working for Children, Living with Children.* Oxford: Heinemann Professional Publishing.

Mayall, B. and Petrie, P. (1983) *Childminding and Day Nurseries: What Kind of Care?* London: Heinemann.

Mayall, B. and Storey, P. (1998) A school health service for children? *Children and Society*, 12(2): 86–97.

Maynard, M. (1994) Methods, practice and epistemology: The debate about feminism and research, in M. Maynard and J. Purvis (eds) *Researching Women's Lives from a Feminist Perspective.* London: Taylor & Francis.

Maynard, M. (1998) Feminists' knowledge and the knowledge of feminisms:

Epistemology, theory, methodology and method, in T. May and M. Williams (eds) *Knowing the Social World*. Buckingham: Open University Press.

Mead, G.H. (1967) *Mind, Self and Society*. Chicago: Chicago University Press.

Meighan, R. (1995) *John Holt: Personalised Education and the Reconstruction of Schooling*. Nottingham: Educational Heretics Press.

Meighan, R. and Siraj-Blatchford, I. (1997) *A Sociology of Educating*. 3rd edn. London: Cassell.

Meyers, D.T. (1997) *Feminist Social Thought: A Reader*. New York: Routledge.

Micklewright, J. and Stewart, K. (2000) *The Welfare of Europe's Children*. Bristol: Policy Press.

Millett, K. (1969) *Sexual Politics*. New York: Avon Books.

Mills, C.W. (1967) *The Sociological Imagination*. Oxford: Oxford University Press.

Mitchell, J. (1971) *Woman's Estate*. Harmondsworth: Penguin.

Mizen, P., Bolton, A. and Pole, C. (1999) School age workers: The paid employment of children in Britain, *Work, Employment and Society*, 13(3): 423–38.

Mizen, P., Pole, C. and Bolton, A. (2001a) Why be a school age worker? in P. Mizen, C. Pole and A. Bolton (eds) *Hidden Hands: International Perspectives on Children's Work and Labour*. London: Falmer.

Mizen, P., Pole, C. and Bolton, A. (eds) (2001b) *Hidden Hands: International Perspectives on Children's Work and Labour*. London: RoutledgeFalmer.

Montandon, C. (2001) The negotiation of influence: Children's experiences of parental education practices in Geneva, in L. Alanen and B. Mayall (eds) *Conceptualizing Child–Adult Relations*. London: RoutledgeFalmer.

Morrow, V. (1994) Responsible children? Aspects of children's work and employment outside school in contemporary UK, in B. Mayall (ed.) *Children's Childhoods: Observed and Experienced*. London: Falmer Press.

Morrow, V. (2000) 'Dirty looks' and 'trampy places' in young people's accounts of community and neighbourhood: Implications for health inequalities, *Critical Public Health*, 10(2): 141–52.

Morss, J. (1990) *The Biologising of Childhood: Developmental Psychology and the Darwinian Myth*. Hove and London: Lawrence Erlbaum Associates.

Moss, P. (1997) Early childhood services in Europe, *Policy Options*, 18(1): 27–30.

Moss, P. (2001) Where next for 'childcare'? *Childcare Now*, 14: 1–4.

National Statistics (2001) *Census 2001*. London: National Statistics.

Newson, J. and Newson, E. (1970) *Four Years Old in an Urban Community*. Harmondsworth: Penguin.

Newson, J. and Newson, E. (1978) *Seven Years Old in the Home Environment*. Harmondsworth: Penguin.

Oakley, A. (1972) *Sex, Gender and Society*. London: Temple Smith.

Oakley, A. (1994) Women and children first and last: parallels and differences between children's and women's studies, in B. Mayall (ed.) *Children's Childhoods: Observed and Experienced*. London: Falmer.

Oakley, A. (2000) *Experiments in Knowing*. Oxford: Blackwell.

Oakley, A. (2002) *Gender on Planet Earth*. Cambridge: Polity Press and New York: New Press.

O'Brien, M. (2000) *Childhood, Urban Space and Citizenship: Child-Sensitive Urban*

Regeneration. Children 5–16 Research Briefing No. 16. Swindon: Economic and Social Research Council.

O'Brien, M., Jones, D., Sloan, D. and Rustin, M. (2000) Children's independent spatial mobility in the urban public realm, *Childhood*, 7(3): 257–78.

O'Donnell, M. and Sharpe, S. (2000) *Uncertain Masculinities: Youth, Ethnicity and Class in Contemporary Britain.* London: Routledge.

Office for National Statistics (1998) *Population Trends 91.* London: Stationery Office.

Office for National Statistics (2000) *Social Trends 2000.* London: Stationery Office.

Oldman, D. (1994) Childhood as a mode of production, in B. Mayall (ed.) *Children's Childhoods: Observed and Experienced.* London: Falmer.

Opie, I. (1993) *The People in the Playground.* Oxford: Oxford University Press.

Opie, I. and Opie, P. (1969) *Children's Games in Street and Playground.* Oxford: Oxford University Press.

Oppenheim, C. and Lister, R. (1996) The politics of child poverty 1979–1995, in J. Pilcher and S. Wagg (eds) *Thatcher's Children: Politics, Childhood and Society in the 1980s and 1990s.* London: Falmer.

Osler, A. (ed.) (2000) *Citizenship and Democracy in Schools: Diversity, Identity, Equality.* Stoke on Trent: Trentham Books.

Ouston, J. and Hood, S. (2000) *Home–School Agreements: A True Partnership?* London: Research and Information on State Education Trust.

Parton, N. (1985) *The Politics of Child Abuse.* London: Macmillan.

Parton, N. (1991) *Governing the Family: Child Care, Child Protection and the State.* London: Macmillan.

Pearson, G. (1983) *Hooligan: A History of Respectable Fears.* London: Macmillan.

Penn, H. (2000) Policy and practice in childcare and nursery education, *Journal of Social Policy*, 29(1): 37–54.

Penn, H. (2001) What does integration mean for children? *Childcare Now*, 14: 3.

Pilcher, J. (1994) Mannheim's sociology of generations: An undervalued legacy, *British Journal of Sociology*, 45(3): 481–95.

Pilcher, J. and Wagg, S. (eds) (1996) *Thatcher's Children: Politics, Childhood and Society in the 1980s and 1990s.* London: Falmer.

Pollard, A., Broadfoot, P., Croll, P., Osborn, M. and Abbott, D. (1994) *Changing English Primary Schools: The Impact of the Education Reform Act at Key Stage One.* London: Cassell.

Polnay, L. (1998) A school health service for children?: A commentary, *Children and Society*, 12(2): 98–100.

Postman, N. (1983) *The Disappearance of Childhood.* London: W.H. Allen.

Pringle, K. (1998) *Children and Social Welfare in Europe.* Buckingham: Open University Press.

Pritchard, M.S. (1996) *Reasonable Children: Moral Education and Moral Learning.* Lawrence, KS: University Press of Kansas.

Prout, A. and James, A. (1990) A new paradigm for the sociology of childhood? Provenance, promise and problems, in A. James and A. Prout (eds) *Constructing and Reconstructing Childhood: Contemporary Issues in the Sociological Study of Childhood.* London: Falmer.

Qvortrup, J. (1985) Placing children in the division of labour, in P. Close and R. Collins (eds) *Family and Economy in Modern Society.* London: Macmillan.

Qvortrup, J. (1991) *Childhood as a Social Phenomenon – An Introduction to a Series of National Reports*, Eurosocial Report 36/1991. Vienna: European Centre.

Qvortrup, J. (1994) Childhood matters: an introduction, in J. Qvortrup, M. Bardy, G. Sgritta and H. Wintersberger (eds) *Childhood Matters: Social Theory, Practice and Politics*. Aldershot: Avebury Press.

Qvortrup, J. (1995) From useful to useful: The historical continuity of children's constructive participation, in P.A. Adler and P. Adler (eds) *Sociological Studies of Children*, Vol. 7. Greenwich, CT: JAI Press.

Qvortrup, J. (2001) School-work, paid work and the changing obligations of childhood, in P. Mizen, C. Pole and A. Bolton (eds) *Hidden Hands: International Perspectives on Children's Work and Labour*. London: Routledge-Falmer.

Qvortrup, J., Bardy, M., Sgritta, G. and Wintersberger, H. (eds) (1994) *Childhood Matters: Social Theory, Practice and Politics*. Aldershot: Avebury Press.

Radcliffe Richards, J. (1980) *The Sceptical Feminist*. Harmondsworth: Penguin.

Rahman, M., Palmer, G., Kenway, P. and Howarth, C. (2000) *Monitoring Poverty and Social Exclusion*. JRF Findings. York: Joseph Rowntree Foundation.

Ramazanoglu, C. (1989) *Feminism and the Contradictions of Oppression*. London: Routledge.

Rassool, N. (1999) Flexible identities: Exploring race and gender issues among a group of immigrant pupils in an inner-city comprehensive school, *British Journal of the Sociology of Education*, 20(1): 23–36.

Reay, D. (1995) A silent majority? Mothers in parental involvement, *Women's Studies International Forum*, 18: 337–48.

Ribbens, J. (1993a) Standing by the school gate – the boundaries of maternal authority, in M. David, R. Edwards, M. Hughes and J. Ribbens (eds) *Mothers and Education: Inside Out?* London: Macmillan.

Ribbens, J. (1993b) Having a word with teacher: Ongoing negotiations across home–school boundaries, in M. David, R. Edwards, M. Hughes and J. Ribbens (eds) *Mothers and Education: Inside Out?* London: Macmillan.

Ribbens, J. (1994) *Mothers and their Children: A Feminist Sociology of Childrearing*. London: Sage.

Ribbens McCarthy, J. (2001) *The Family Lives of Young People*. York: Joseph Rowntree Foundation.

Ribbens McCarthy, J., Edwards, R. and Gillies, R. (2000) *Parenting and Step-Parenting: Contemporary Moral Tales*. Centre for Family and Household Research Occasional Paper 4. Oxford: Oxford Brookes University.

Richards, C. (1998) The primary school curriculum: Changes, challenges, questions, in C. Richards and P.H. Taylor (eds) *How Shall We School Our Children? Primary Education and its Future*. London: Falmer.

Riesman, P. (1992) *First Find Your Child a Good Mother*. New Brunswick, NJ: Rutgers University Press.

Robinson, J. (1963) A model of accumulation, in J. Robinson (ed.) *Essays in the Theory of Economic Growth*. London: Macmillan.

Rogers, G. and Standing G. (1981) *Child Work, Poverty and Underdevelopment*. Geneva: International Labour Organisation.

Rogoff, B. (1990) *Apprenticeship in Thinking: Cognitive Development in Social Context*. New York: Oxford University Press.

Rowbotham, S. (1973) *Woman's Consciousness, Man's World*. Harmondsworth: Penguin.

Rutter, J. (1994) *Refugee Children in the Classroom*. Stoke on Trent: Trentham Books.

Ryder, N. (1965) The cohort as a concept in the study of social change, *American Sociological Review*, 30: 843–61.

Sainsbury, D. (ed.) (1994a) *Gendering Welfare States*. London: Sage.

Sainsbury, D. (1994b) Women's and men's social rights: Gendering dimensions of welfare states, in D. Sainsbury (ed.) *Gendering Welfare States*. London: Sage.

Salmi, M. (1996) *Combining Work and Family in Finnish Family Policy*. Finland: Ministry for Foreign Affairs.

Sandbaek, M. (1999) Children with problems: Focusing on everyday life, *Children and Society*, 13(2): 106–18.

Saporiti, A. and Sgritta, G. (1990) *Childhood as a Social Phenomenon: National Report Italy*. Eurosocial Report 36/2. Vienna: European Centre.

Save the Children (1995) *Towards a Children's Agenda: New Challenges for Social Development*. London: Save the Children.

Scarre, G. (ed.) (1989a) *Children, Parents and Politics*. Cambridge: Cambridge University Press.

Scarre, G. (1989b) Justice between generations, in G. Scarre (ed.) *Children, Parents and Politics*. Cambridge: Cambridge University Press.

Scott, S. (2000) The Impact of Risk and Parental Risk Anxiety on the Everyday Worlds of Children. Children 5–16 Research Briefing, No. 19. Swindon: Economic and Social Research Council.

Scraton, P. (ed.) (1997) *'Childhood' in 'Crisis'?* London: UCL Press.

Segal, L. (1995) A feminist looks at the family, in J. Muncie, M. Wetherell, R. Dallos and A. Cochrane (eds) *Understanding the Family*. London: Sage.

Segal, L. (1999) *Why Feminism?: Gender, Psychology, Politics*. Cambridge: Polity Press.

Shier, H. (2001) Pathways to participation: Openings, opportunities and obligations, *Children and Society*, 15(2): 107–17.

Shweder, R.A., Mahapatra, M. and Miller, J.G. (1986) Culture and moral development, in J. Kagan and S. Lamb (eds) *The Emergence of Morality in Young Children*. Chicago, IL: University of Chicago Press.

Silva, E.B and Smart, C. (1999) *The New Family?* London: Sage.

Simon, B. (1988) *Bending the Rules: The Baker 'Reform' of Education*. London: Lawrence and Wishart.

Simonen, L. and Kovalainen, A. (1998) Paradoxes of social care restructuring: The Finnish case, in J. Lewis (ed.) *Gender, Social Care and Welfare State Restructuring in Europe*. Aldershot: Ashgate.

Sinclair, R. (ed.) (1996) Special issue on research with children, *Children and Society*, 10(2).

Sipilä, J. (ed.) (1997) *Social Care Services: The Key to Scandinavian Welfare Models*. Aldershot: Ashgate.

Sluckin, A. (1981) *Growing up in the Playground*. London: Routledge and Kegan Paul.

Smart, C. and Neale, B. (2000a) *Post Divorce Childhoods: Perspectives from*

Children. Research Briefing, University of Leeds: Centre for Research on Family, Kinship and Childhood.

Smart, C. and Neale, B. (2000b) *New Childhoods: Co-parenting After Divorce.* Children 5–16 Research Briefing No. 7. Swindon: Economic and Social Research Council.

Smith, A., Gollop, M., Marshall, K. and Nairn, K. (eds) (2000) *Advocating for Children: International Perspectives on Children's Rights*. Dunedin, NZ: University of Otago Press.

Smith, D. (1974) Women, the family and corporate capitalism, in M.L. Stephensen (ed.) *Women in Canada*. Toronto: New Press.

Smith, D. (1988) *The Everyday World as Problematic: Towards a Feminist Sociology*. Milton Keynes: Open University Press.

Smith, D. (1999) *Writing the Social: Critique, Theory and Investigations*. Toronto: University of Toronto Press.

Smith, F. and Barker, J. (2000) Contested spaces: Children's experiences of out of school care in England and Wales, *Childhood*, 7(3): 315–34.

Smith, R. (2000) Whose childhood? The politics of homework, *Children and Society*, 14(4): 316–25.

Solberg, A. (1990) Negotiating childhood: changing constructions of age for Norwegian children, in A. James and A. Prout (eds) *Constructing and Reconstructing Childhood: Contemporary Issues in the Sociological Study of Childhood*. London: Falmer.

Song, M. (1997) Children's labour in ethnic family businesses: The case of Chinese take-aways in Britain, *Ethnic and Racial Studies*, 20(4): 690–716.

Stacey, M. (1976) The health service consumer: A sociological misconception, in M. Stacey (ed.) *The Sociology of the NHS*, Sociological Review Monograph no. 22. Keele: University of Keele.

Stacey, M. (1981) The division of labour revisited, or overcoming the two Adams, in P. Abrams, R. Deem, J. Finch and P. Roch (eds) *Practice and Progress in British Sociology 1950–1980*. London: Allen and Unwin.

Stacey, M. and Davies, C. (1983) Division of labour in child health care: Final report to the Social Science Research Council. Unpublished report, University of Warwick.

Standing, K. (1999a) Lone mothers and parental involvement: A contradiction in policy, *Journal of Social Policy*, 28: 479–96.

Steedman, C. (1988) The mother made conscious: The historical development of a primary school pedagogy, in M. Woodhead and A. McGrath (eds) *Family, School and Society*. London: Hodder and Stoughton.

Stephens, S. (1993) Children at risk: Constructing social problems and policies. An essay book review, *Childhood*, 1(4): 246–51.

Stock, B. (1994) *Health and Safety in Schools*. London: Croner Publications Limited.

Sutton-Smith, B. (ed.) (1979) *Play and Learning*. New York: Gardner Press.

Taskinen, S. (1996) Finland, in J. Ditch, H. Barnes and J. Bradshaw (eds) *Developments in National Family Policies in 1995*. York: Social Policy Research Unit.

Therborn, G. (1993) Children's rights since the constitution of modern childhood: A comparative study of western nations, in J. Qvortrup (ed.) *Childhood as a Social Phenomenon: Lessons from an International Project.* Report 47/1993. Vienna: European Centre.

Therborn, G. (1996) Child politics: Dimensions and perspectives, *Childhood*, 3(1): 29–44.

Thomson, R., Holland, J., Henderson, S., McGrellis, S. and Sharpe, S. (2000) Researching childhood: Time, memory and method. Paper presented to the British Sociological Association Annual Conference, York, 17–20 April.

Thorne, B. (1987) Re-visioning women: Where are the children? *Gender and Society*, 1(1): 85–109.

Thorne, B. (1993) *Gender Play: Girls and Boys at School.* New Brunswick, NJ: Rutgers University Press.

Toynbee, P. and Walker, D. (2001) *Did Things Get Better? An Audit of Labour's Success and Failures.* Harmondsworth: Penguin.

Triggs, P. and Pollard, A. (1998) Pupil experience and a curriculum for life-long learning, in C. Richards and P.H. Taylor (eds) *How Shall We School Our Children? Primary Education and its Future.* London: Falmer.

United Kingdom (1999) *Convention on the Rights of the Child: Second Report to the UN Committee on the Rights of the Child by the United Kingdom.* London: Stationery Office.

United Nations (1989) *Convention on the Rights of the Child.* Geneva: United Nations.

United Nations Children's Fund (1998) *The Human Rights of Women and Children: Challenges and Opportunities.* Stockholm: Rädda Barnen.

United Nations Children's Fund (2001) *A League Table of Child Deaths by Injury in Rich Nations.* Innocenti Report Card No. 2. Florence, Italy: UNICEF Innocenti Research Centre.

United Nations Development Fund for Women (2000) *Progress of the World's Women.* New York: United Nations Development Fund for Women.

Urwin, C. and Sharland, E. (1992) From bodies to minds in childcare literature: Advice to parents in inter-war Britain, in R. Cooter (ed.) *In the Name of the Child: Health and Welfare 1880–1940.* London: Routledge.

Valentine, G. (1996) Angels and devils: moral landscapes of childhood, *Environment and Planning D: Society and Space*, 14: 581–99.

Valentine, G. (1999) 'Oh please, Mum. Oh please, Dad': Negotiating children's spatial boundaries, in L. McKie, S. Bowlby and S. Gregory (eds) *Gender, Power and the Household.* London: Macmillan.

Valentine, G., Holloway, S.L. and Bingham, N. (2000) Transforming cyberspace: Children's interventions in the new public sphere, in S.L. Holloway and G. Valentine (eds) *Children's Geographies: Playing, Living Learning.* London: Routledge.

Verhellen, E. (1993) Children and participation rights, in P.-L. Heiliö, E. Lauronen and M. Bardy (eds) *Politics of Childhood and Children at Risk.* Eurosocial Report 45/1993. Vienna: European Centre.

Vincent, C. and Warren, S. (2000) Education for motherhood? in C. Vincent, *Including Parents? Education, Citizenship and Parental Agency.* Buckingham: Open University Press.

von Hirsch, E. (1998) Rearing children to be moral agents, in J. La Fontaine and

H. Rydstrøm (eds) *The Invisibility of Children*, working papers on childhood and the study of children. Linköping, Sweden: Department of Child Studies, Linköping University.

Waksler, F.C. (ed.) (1991) *Studying the Social Worlds of Children: Sociological Readings*. London: Falmer.

Walden, G. (1996) *We Should Know Better: Bridging the Education Crisis*. London: Fourth Estate.

Walkerdine, V. and Lucey, H. (1989) *Democracy in the Kitchen: Regulating Mothers and Socialising Daughters*. London: Virago.

Ward, C. (1978) *The Child in the City*. London: Architectural Press.

Ward, C. (1988) *The Child in the Country*. London: Robert Hale Limited.

Watson, N. (2000) *Lives of Disabled Children*. Children 5–16 Research Briefing No. 8. Swindon: Economic and Social Research Council.

Williamson, H. and Butler, I. (1995) No-one ever listens to us: Interviewing children and young people, in C. Cloke and M. Davies (eds) *Participation and Empowerment in Child Protection*. Chichester: John Wiley.

Wilson, C. (1995) Issues for children and young people in local authority accommodation, in C. Cloke and M. Davies (eds) *Participation and Empowerment in Child Protection*. Chichester: John Wiley.

Wilson, E. (1977) *Women and the Welfare State*. London: Tavistock.

Woodhead, M. (1997) Psychology and the cultural construction of children's needs, in A. James and A. Prout (eds) *Constructing and Reconstructing Childhood: Contemporary Issues in the Sociological Study of Childhood*. 2nd edn. London: Falmer.

Woodhead, M., Faulkner, D. and Littleton, K. (eds) (1998) *Cultural Worlds of Early Childhood*. London: Routledge.

Wyness, M. (2000) *Contesting Childhood*. London: Falmer.

Young, M. and Whitty, G. (eds) (1977) *Society, State and Schooling*. Lewes: Falmer.

Zelizer, V. (1985) *Pricing the Priceless Child: The Changing Social Value of Children*. New York: Basic Books.

Index

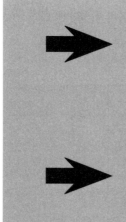